THE JOURNEY
Coping with Loved Ones in the Strange World of Dementia

Myrtle Sobers

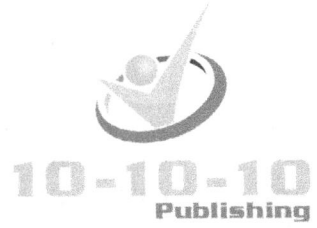

10-10-10
Publishing

Contents

In memory of my dearly loved mother,
Victoria Baptiste

Acknowledgments

I would like to thank ...

My sisters, Shirley Meridin and Hazel Leeyaw, for their encouragement to tell my story.

Lori Murphy and Jennifer Le, from the Raymond Aaron group, for their support and guidance.

Foreword

This book reveals a very personal and subjective response to the changing patterns of behaviour of a very dear loved one that suffered from Alzheimer's disease. It is helpful and informative particularly to families who are similarly affected. It teaches: what to anticipate, how to deal with feelings of fear, what uncertainties we must overcome, how to hold on to a positive attitude, and what signs and symptoms are associated with this disorder. It makes clear that love, patience and understanding are essential and indispensable ingredients for the acceptance and proper handling of this most emotionally painful illness. The book will be of enormous help and support not only to affected families but to caregivers as well.

Alzheimer's disease is a primary degenerative brain disease of unknown etiology which is insidious in onset and associated with gradual but progressive deterioration leading to death in an average time of ten years. It is the most common form of dementia, and may have an onset in middle age or earlier but the incidence is higher in later life. The associated genetic defects as well as the relevant neurochemical changes are quite well mapped out. There are well-documented familial cases, some following an autosomal-dominant pattern of inheritance with linkage to either chromosome 19 or 21. Patients with a family history of Alzheimer's, those with Down's syndrome (trisomy 21) and those who've had head injuries are particularly at risk.

Even though much is known about the clinical features, the neurochemical changes, the genetics and general pathophysiology of Alzheimer's disease, a definitive pharmacologic cure has not yet been found. Nevertheless, the physician's role in treating the patient and family remains vital. He must discontinue all nonessential medications and treat all associated illnesses or developments. He should guide and support the family through the course of the disease and facilitate community services as needed. Support groups such as Alzheimer's Associations often are of value to the family in clarifying and helping them to anticipate problems. Signs of patient abuse by an overstressed caregiver should be watched for. Legal counsel should be recommended to help the patient and family devise plans for ongoing management and ultimate disposition of assets needed.

The onset of disruptive behaviour should always prompt a search for a new illness or additional medication. Exacerbation of cognitive dysfunction may occur with a mild infection, with therapeutic levels of a number of drugs, with non-prescribed drugs, with alcohol or as a result of electrolyte imbalance or urinary retention.

It seems clear that the author's misconceptions concerning her mother's dementia led to much confusion, frustration and hurt. *"Misinformed, we thought her disease could be fixed."*

Perhaps because of this book others will come to a better understanding of this dreaded disease and learn how best to cope if confronted with it.

Keith A. Forde, MD

About the Author

I am a caregiver at a long-term care facility. This was a path carved out for me it would seem like, by faith. I had no interest in nursing. I remember my mother would say, she could see me as a nurse, and often referred to me as such. She would affectionately call me her nurse, as I would often attend to friends who suffered minor injuries while at play, even if I was too young to understand it all. As I grew older, I did not care to witness the distress on the faces of those who were suffering, and on the ones who were suffering along with them.

My background is in administration and, after eighteen years in that profession, I found myself in the field of nursing. I came to like it. As a nurse I provided caring, comforting, cheering and, to my surprise, counselling, even if it is not in my job description, which made me appreciate and value the tasks I had been given. I found myself filled with compassion for the people I served and cared for, even if this is not the primary expectation of my role. When a resident smiled and said "I love you," it made what I do every day worthwhile.

Then it occurred to me that this path for nursing was no accident and, in fact, was a course carved out by some divine intervention. This then became clear when my mother, Victoria, was afflicted with Alzheimer's disease and dementia. My mother exhibited all the symptoms, including loss of memory, judgement, and reasoning, and changes in mood and behaviour. It is worth noting that dementia is an umbrella term for a variety of brain disorders; within that, Alzheimer's is the most common.

My siblings and I went through the cycles of grief and guilt associated with this discovery. We felt guilty that we could not help her to get better. We were not directly told that she had Alzheimer's, nor were we educated or informed on how best to provide care. The doctor, despite his knowledge of how the disease progressed, was not forthcoming with the facts or advice. Misinformed, we thought her disease could be fixed. We were suffused with anger because, every day, she behaved differently, as if she was a different person, and we had to relearn daily how to cope. For example, she would always insist on visiting someone who we knew was not around. We got angry with her for not being normal. We got angry with each other because the burden of care meant we could no longer live normal lives. We were vigilant to keep her safe, and this took a toll on our families and wellbeing. What we did not know was that, because of the nature of the disease, she could not understand or control her behaviour. It was slowly becoming clear to us that this was not a mental breakdown that could be controlled with medication.

That obviously was not the case. Then we felt fear. We feared that she might never return to her normal self and, of course, she never did. There were many times she got annoyed with us for trying to protect her from herself. We loved her too much to see her tormented like that. My mother was only 5'1" and, before the disease took its ugly toll on her, was a vibrant and vivacious woman. She loved working and shopping, and cooking and cleaning. All her children towered over her in stature, yet she commanded our attention, especially when it came to disciplining us. She was also light hearted and lots of fun to be around. She was a seemingly healthy person, who loved life and her four children and grandchildren.

Yet once her deterioration began, all those memories had to be boxed up. We had to be firm and we had to care. We felt ashamed at times at her unexpected outbursts, which could happen anytime, in front of friends or strangers. We kept her in the house. This bothers me to this day, and I live daily with the guilt.

My mother's behaviour was turbulent and chaotic. There were episodes of bitterness, periods of loneliness, and frequent bouts of confusion. She was an active woman and insisted on moving at all times. This disrupted our sleep, so we took turns caring for her so that each of us could get a break. It was hard work, and our stress was compounded by the realization that we did not know what to do or how to cope. But in the end, we fell back on the easiest and simplest thing we could; we returned to the most fundamental value that was instilled in all of us, and that was to love. We loved her no matter what.

About the Author

My sisters and our respective families experienced firsthand the initial shock, denial, and emotional rollercoaster of loving someone with dementia, my mother.

This book is written as a simple and short guide to lend support to families, friends, and caregivers of individuals diagnosed with this debilitating illness. I deeply empathize with what you are going through, having experienced first-hand the countless emotional, psychological, social, spiritual, and financial challenges that anyone on this path will encounter. The first five chapters chart my personal journey, and that of my siblings, in taking care of our mother. I have attempted in portions to depict the world as she saw it when gripped in the inescapable claws of the disease. By doing it this way, I hope you will come to understand the fragmented and broken reality that she faced, and that you may have more compassion for your loved one who is now suffering. In subsequent chapters, I share clinical advice and experiences.

If in some way this book, by mapping the way forward, can bring you a little comfort, a little relief, and a little help to regain some control over your life, it will have done its job admirably.

Introduction

I wrote this book with love and compassion for patients with dementia, and for all the caregivers, family, and friends who undergo the daily routines of caring and kindness. I see the unstinting devotion to the task at hand, every day, at the long-term care facility where I work. This book is meant for those in connection with loved ones and the caregivers of those inflicted with the disorder of dementia. It is meant to give a simple and yet powerful understanding of the caring necessity to cope with this unexpected and traumatic turn of events, and the strategies and skills related to the long-term care of the loved one suffering from dementia.

Alzheimer's is said to be the most common form of dementia. This progressive and degenerative brain disease is characterized by the irreversible loss of brain cells. Alzheimer's disease affects memory, reasoning ability, and brings about the inability to make proper judgment, or identify objects and people. The symptoms get progressively worse and, in the more advanced stages, the patient is unable to carry out daily functioning activities. This causes anxiety for the patient and family member who must deal with the progressive decline brought about by the disease. The reality of the disease cleaves your world and that of the patient, and nothing will ever be the same again. I have written this as an easy go-to book for family and friends who need a quick reference or tips on coping strategies. Having personally gone through the shock of the diagnosis, the continual pain of wanting to do more but not being able to do enough, and having suffered a deeply personal loss, I write this so that others may have an easier time through their own journeys. However, the book is not only focused on the mechanics of coping. In writing the book, I have also thought of all the friends, relatives, and immediate family who, in one way or another, are irreversibly touched and affected by the disease.

You have overcome the initial fear that surged in your body after you heard the diagnosis for your loved one. Painful as it is, you haven't run away. You have searched for the best medical team and have settled on a plan of action. You have maintained your composure and realized that you are not alone. However, you may still be feeling disconnected from reality and, unknowingly, you are transferring this feeling to your loved one, the one who is undergoing the irreversible changes.

This sense of dislocation is understandable. The period between first finding out the news and making the appropriate adjustments is never easy for anyone, no matter how tightly knit the family is. Your lives have been upturned and will never be the same. As the caregiver or the onlooker, emotions such as anger, frustration and the feeling of victimization – "why me?" – will bubble up and erode the bonds of family and love with the patient. Accept that these feelings are natural, but also understand that love came first, and love helps you stay connected. Remember the happy and joyful times you had before this unwelcome intruder invaded your home. Remember your mother, father, husband, brother, sister or friend the way they were. Those memories are your touchstone to hope; they are your connection to the laughter you shared. The recollections of times well spent remind you that life goes on. It may not proceed as you had hoped or dreamt of, but life will and must continue. Love sheds light on dark fears, and drives those shadows away.

Amidst the feelings of despair, anxiety, frustration, and disconnection, grasp on to the moments when your brain comes across a memory of laughter. The person you shared this precious time with is the same person who is before you; it's just that you will be creating different and new types of memories from now on. My own mother would react with delight at the birds and flowers when we took her outside, as if she were seeing them for the first time. She would turn her face to the breeze to enjoy its soft touch. Her face would break out into a broad smile that was simple and priceless to us. Her smile revived all memories of what she was—all the laughter, all those funny times we had together, came flooding back to me. I know those times cannot be retrieved, but at least I have those memories. As a more recent example, I would like to share an experience that I had with one of my residents at the nursing home. Let me call her Jane.

As I wrote this book, I was always on the lookout for inspiration. But I did not expect that it would come from Jane.

Jane exhibits the behaviour typical of dementia. She is in her eighties and is a quiet, anti-social person who stays in her room most of the time. "Hi Jane, how are you today?" And the answer that would unfailingly shoot back to me was, "What do you want? Get out of here!" I would reply, "Jane, you know I love you, so let's get this done," and I would go on my way. We would play out this ritual each and every time I entered the room. I would smile when I approached her and would be greeted with the same angry response: "Hurry up and get out." One day, I went in to hand her a glass of water, and expected Jane to behave as she always did. This day, she caught me by surprise. She looked up at me, made eye contact, and said, "You know that you are one of the nicest people that come in here." Tears rimmed my eyes; this appreciation coming from a woman who had, without fail, been unwelcoming of me every day. It is for these people that I write this book. I said to her, hoping that she was still in a state of clarity, "I will cherish this moment for as long as I can remember it." I share this with you so that you may know that somewhere in that stranger who sits or stands before you, is the person you love.

This book explores the responsibility to connect with your loved ones, no matter what happens, and no matter how nasty the interactions may be. The disease is not their fault, and it is not your fault either. Accept the circumstances for what they are, and find the courage to move beyond the diagnosis. It may take a lot of adjusting on your end, but take care to rise above the fear and fill your thoughts with love and compassion.

Alzheimer's can strike randomly with or without a genetic predisposition. Whatever the reason, once it arrives, it changes lives irreversibly. As a caregiver in nursing, I chose to write this book to give hope to families of patients in all stages of the illness. Those struck by Alzheimer's disease, and other forms of dementia, lose most or all of their reasoning abilities. Sometimes we think they know exactly what they are doing or saying and we behave or react to them as if they are in full possession of their faculties, but they aren't. As the caregiver, it is natural to feel trapped as the disease progresses. This is a path you've never traveled before, and there will be times when you don't know how to relate, when interactions become difficult and, on occasion, impossible. Frustration will get the better of you, but don't let it swamp you for the entire length of the journey. You need to be wholeheartedly present for the loved one, the patient, for the remaining span of his or her life. There are no two ways about it. But think about this: When the loved one moves on, will you be able to say that you did whatever you could?

I encourage all caregivers, family, and friends to constantly and consistently work on establishing a strong connection with the patient. Somehow, sometime, somewhere, like the raindrops on a parched ground, the connection will be felt, cherished, and treasured, even if for the most fleeting of moments. Participate with them in events, interact through activities that I describe in this book, and join them in their exercises. This is a way of building a bridge into their world, and to creating a deep, meaningful, long-lasting relationship. Even if there are times when you are strangers to each other, there are pursuits and events you can both enjoy that have an impact on your lives.

My hope for writing this book is that all of us recognize that individuals afflicted with dementia, or more specifically Alzheimer's disease, are a part of our lives. If the patient is a parent, remember that he or she once nurtured you, loved you, and guided you. I encourage you to connect with your loved ones in positive ways, not from anger or frustration or helplessness, but in life-affirming, life-reinforcing, and life-expanding ways. If there are any opportunities when you can stay in the present moment, step away from judgment and meet them halfway in their strange world, by loving and recognizing them for who they are, even if they cannot reciprocate; those are moments of gold. By truly, meaningfully, and wholeheartedly reaching out and connecting with them, you are enriching their connection with life, no matter how tenuous it may seem to you, while simultaneously adding depth, texture, and dimension to your own life. I know, from my own experience and from my work, it is an immensely tough journey. But truly, truly let me resort to an age-worn saying: Love really does conquer all.

Chapter -1-

The Mystery of Dementia

"A good head and a good heart are always a formidable combination."
Nelson Mandela

This story references dementia (a group of symptoms) and Alzheimer's (the disease). It provides a no-nonsense look into what general changes of an Alzheimer's disease patient and the inability to remember things and to do normal activities look like.

The Onset of Dementia

Mom:

It has been four years since I visited with my brother. He called me yesterday and invited me to come over next Saturday. I am sure that's what he said. We talked and laughed like old times. I enjoyed every moment we spent talking. It brought back good old childhood memories. He is my brother; we grew up to-gether. I think of him all the time. I am happy to go on this visit, even though it's a long journey. His wife cooks up nice gourmet food, and I must go to enjoy some good food. Oh! Did my son call today? He calls every day and talks to me. I am confused; I cannot remember if this call was from my son or my brother.

Lately, my memory is not so good. I must ask my son to buy me some brain tonic. I've worked very hard, ever since I was a teenager. I raised my four kids and took care of my husband. That phone call still lingers on my mind. I don't know what to do. I must call my son, to ask if he called. I know I have the phone number somewhere, but I forget where I put it. I have been looking for the past few minutes. It was in a book; I wrote it down myself. This must be old age, but I am in my mid-sixties; I should not be having this memory loss problem, and it's getting worse. I am forgetting where I placed things and have poor recall of new information and occurrences. I forget so quickly. I brought this to the attention of my family, but they dismissed the symptoms and attributed them to other reasons such as stress. They say I am thinking too much about many things, so they don't take me seriously. Well, I am going to see my brother anyway; I have not seen him in a long time. I can't sit here and wait around; I'm leaving now.

Oftentimes, in the initial stages of Alzheimer's disease, the warning signs that something is wrong are usually ignored by the family, as there are no obvious symptoms. If you notice changes in yourself or a loved one, even if they seem minor, get tested. Make sure there is no physical damage that is leading to these uncomfortable and inconvenient changes, such as memory lapses. By delaying the process, you place yourself or your loved one in further jeopardy, if there is a disease. Deeper and irreversible damage is being done by failing to get it diagnosed in a timely fashion.

The Family – Dawning of Awareness

*"Everything that irritates us about others can lead us
to an understanding of ourselves."*
Carl Jung

It was the inability and inconsistency in performing any normal task that alerted our family to the possibility that something was not right. The gradual memory loss gained momentum, and it was impossible for our mother to grasp difficult concepts. It took two years for her children to recognize that this behaviour was not just an aging problem; it was far worse than what we imagined.

The disorientation, impaired judgment, personality changes, and even the inability to speak in fluent sentences, were increasingly challenging. She frequently hallucinated, and she was constantly confused about what was or wasn't in her presence. She would confront the imaginary object or person by shouting contentious arguments and conjured revenge. Alzheimer's disease also affects a part of the brain called the amygdala, which controls fear and anger. This area of the brain, when affected, results in diminished judgment and irrepressible emotional responses, which leads to outbursts of temper and violent reactions.

The parietal lobes and temporal lobes suffer as well. The results of these are rapid deterioration of cognitive skills, such as reading and writing abilities, maths skills, and space perception. Those with affected temporal lobes also become unable to find objects. Language capabilities, recognition of familiar things, people, and places or even remembering personal information, slowly disappears. My mother exhibited all of the above symptoms. It was difficult for us to comprehend her dilemma, without a scope on the disease. Whatever window of coherence left within my mother's brain was too small for any rational assumption. We had to make the decisions that would help us to reach the appropriate treatment for our peace and her safety.

In earlier years, when medicine was less informed about dementia, such symptoms were thought to indicate senility. To be senile is to exhibit a loss of cognitive abilities such as memory, associated with old age. The growing recognition among family members that something was wrong was accompanied by increasing frustration and helplessness. She was behaving so strangely, at times, that we thought she was mad, and it seemed impossible for us to handle these nasty changes in behaviour.

We shouted at her to smarten up or else we would leave the house. We yelled, "You are a mad person; stop acting that way," and were visibly shaken that the vibrant, wonderful woman we knew was disappearing. We tried to get her to cooperate, despite her perplexing state of mind, as we scrambled for answers. There was a stand-off between the uncooperative mom and her bewildered adult children, and the arguments stacked up and continued. Even in her irrational and confused state, our mother was able to sense the waves of frustration and anger that were peeling off her kids. She was frightened and worried, and turned combative. Suddenly, someone decided she had enough, and the noise dialled down. As if struck by divine intervention, we backed away, deep in remorse for shouting at our mother. It was the defining moment. We apologized, quietly, in tears, or held ourselves stoically.

One by one, we approached her slowly and calmly, presenting composed tranquil demeanors. Our mother was still distrusting but, as each of us drew closer, we encouraged her to sit with us. Each of us said, gently, "I love you, Mom." Each affirmation was followed by a moment of silence; then another would reaffirm, "I love you."

Our mother did not immediately relax but, with each calm statement of love, she finally settled, slowly trusting that her children would not, inexplicably, yell or be angry with her. The family siblings took deep breaths, stayed quiet and, within minutes, she was asleep in her chair.

Dementia had irrevocably and completely changed this woman, her moods, and personality. Disruptive behaviour and other problems were surfacing.

Another year would go by before the family made the brave decision to have a comprehensive diagnosis. It would take twelve more months of repeated moments like this one before we would acknowledge that perhaps our mother was suffering from a degenerative brain condition.

The person with dementia is very sensitive to what you are feeling. They do not understand the difference between verbal sarcasm and the truth. People with dementia rely heavily on the feelings that accompany the words. If you are frustrated or angry and intolerant, that feeling is conveyed to the person with dementia, who in turn will react to the negative, and will turn uncooperative and combative.

Getting Ready Through the Lens of Dementia

"For him who has conquered the mind, the mind is the best of friends;
but for one who has failed to do so,
his mind will remain the greatest enemy."
Bhagavad-Gita

Mom:

I think it was my brother who called today. I have not heard from him for a long time. I will get ready to go and visit with him. It's quite a distance to travel, but I will get there somehow. I know my son will take me there. I will have to leave before my daughters get home. They are too protective of me. I know that they love me, but I am an adult and can take care of myself. I raised them; now they want to tell me what to do. I have to get going and stop thinking too much. I am not sure what day it is today, and the time just doesn't seem right. I have a lot to do; I must get ready. I know what I have to do, but why can't I remember what to do next?

I go to the shower; I come out with the washcloth in my hands, and I don't remember what to do with it. I think I should shower, but I am dressed now. Maybe I'll shower later. Maybe I need to pack some clothes. There is a suitcase in the closet; it's just perfect for my trip.

Did my son call today? He calls every day. I must tell him I am going on this journey to visit with my brother. I'm getting more and more anxious. I cannot remember where my brother lives. Things will seem clearer when I leave the house. Nice day; it must be early. I don't know the time, but I am heading out. What is he doing standing at the gate? There is a tall man dressed in black pants and white shirt on the walkway toward the gate. He is staring at me with this mean look on his face. I yell at him to get off my property, but he ignores me. I have to see to it that he leaves before I can leave.

Here comes Sandra; she is a friend of the family. She looks out for me all the time. She is a good woman; she smiles and treats me well.

"I heard you screaming, so I came to see what was wrong," she asks.

"It is that man by the gate," I say as I point.

"What man?" Sandra asks.

"That one. Yes, he is out to get me."

"I don't see anyone. Go back inside until your daughters come home." Sandra tries to persuade me.

"I am going to visit with my brother. He is getting up in age and maybe not doing too good, which is a pity. He was asking me these strange questions, over and over again. He thinks I am losing my mind. He had to be teasing me. I must go and see if everything is all right with him," I tell her.

"Doesn't he live far away?"

"Yes. But I will go out and catch a bus. I have a little money on me that will do until I get there; he will loan me some more. Just follow me to the next corner. I will be alright; I can take care of myself," I tell Sandra.

The person with dementia is deeply appreciative of the simplest of acts such as listening attentively or demonstrating concern, without judgement. The conversations he or she has with a real or imaginary person may be triggered by suppressed memories coming to the surface. They may feel pain or turbulent emotions. Listening patiently to them, regardless of how much of a mumbo-jumbo or how incoherent the dialogue may be, provides them with an opportunity to release these emotions.

The Family Intervention

"In this life we cannot always do great things.
But we can do small things with great love."
Mother Teresa

We panicked when our mother did not come home. We first thought she was with her friend, Sandra, but when darkness fell and 10pm came around, it became apparent that something had to be done, and fast. Incidents like these had to be stopped.

We paired up, bracing ourselves for a more thorough search, and were about to leave when a police car with flashing lights drew up to the gate. Two police officers walked our mother to the door. Emotions ran high and were let loose. The family was understandably sad and upset. This lovely, vibrant woman, now in her early seventies, was exhibiting all the symptoms of Alzheimer's disease. At that time, even from a doctor's point of view and after a medical exam, Alzheimer's wasn't the diagnosis that was handed to us.

However, it was apparent that a severe disease had taken over this woman, and life for all would never be the same. My brother and sisters and I got together to decide what the next steps should be. Mingled with the indecision about our next steps was the confusion about the full extent of our mother's illness.

Our mother, still physically active, would not let anything or anyone stop her from getting to where she wanted to go. She was always seeing an imagined someone and afraid of an unreal something, but would be clever enough to escape them at any cost. There were the men in the television that disliked her, and those at the gate that were out to get her.

We had to take steps to keep her safe—decisions that she would not like. We had to be sure she was getting everything that she needed to be healthy. Even though she insisted there was nothing wrong with her, she cooperated enough with us to visit a psychiatrist. However, getting her to take her medication was a challenge as she firmly believed that she was not sick. These medications made her delusions and anxiety go away.

We knew she would not get better, but medication restored a degree of tranquility to the house and to the family. At this stage of dementia, our mother was easily confused about where she was, and did not remember important information such as her address, phone number, or even the day of the week. She was no longer able to tell time.

At the clinic, the psychiatrist advised us to take care of our own mental and emotional health. We were now embarked on a long-term vigil of care, and each of us had to be in prime mental and physical health to give our mother, now a patient, the right attention and care needed. This relentless disease would slowly take its toll.

It was hard to come to grips with the fact that, with Alzheimer's, there was no going back. There was no rewinding of the clock, nor was there time to stand still. In fact, there is no map on what to do next as this disease progresses. The whole family dynamics was forever altered.

Interventions are best directed toward the interpersonal and physical environments. These changes improve the sense of control that the family, as caregivers, will have. In our case, doors and the outside gate were modified to make it difficult for our mother to leave without us knowing. Changes were made to the lighting, stove, and fridge. The most important job was to create a calm environment that reduced her anxiety and agitation. As the television was a source of agitation, it had to be moved out. The radio had to be put away to reduce excess noise; knives and medications were locked up to keep her safe.

Although those with dementia have much in common in terms of the symptoms, each individual lives out a different storyline. The journey of the patient with dementia is colored and directed by the person's personality traits and life history. We, as caregivers, must provide these precious individuals with love and gentle but firm direction. The direction must be based on a deep understanding of their unique journeys as the disease unfolds. The caregiver must be aware of and stay flexible enough to adjust to the changing needs of the patient, as the dementia progresses.

The Struggle to Leave the House

"Remembering is a great invention of the mind, and if you try hard enough, you can remember anything, whether it really happened or not."
Rodman Philbrick

Mom:

This seems like a new day. I will have my breakfast and go on my journey. I started getting ready yesterday. I have been busy all morning preparing, but I don't seem to be anywhere close to where I need to be. I wait for my son to get back to drive me to my brother's place. He has a car, and I do not need to take the bus. The sun is beginning to dwindle, so it must be about midday, or thereafter. Someone is standing there, observing my every move; he chooses not to assist me for this journey. Why is he not helping me?

I need to get my suitcase into the car. "Come on, take my suitcase to your vehicle," I shout. I am working myself up to anger. Keep calm, I tell myself. But the urge to keep going is strong, and the voices are telling me that I will be running late.

It's drawing near to evening, and the weather is getting cool. I pull from my closet a thick sweater and hat. The voice in my head says that it's cold, so I must be prepared. I am on this journey all by myself, and I must find a way out. I must call my son to help me find my way to the garage. There is a telephone on the wall in the room where I last was. I must be confused and disoriented; why am I seeing things, and why am I unable to leave the house?

I use the phone in the kitchen to call my son, but the numbers are a complete mess. Is someone playing tricks on me? I open the back door, which leads into another part of the house. I make another unsuccessful attempt to call my son. I grab my suitcase and start down a set of stairs that will take me to the back of the house. I try the doors; they will not open for me. I wonder if my son called today. It seems logical to rest for the night, but I cannot sleep, I cannot rest. I keep wondering why it is so difficult for me to find the exit. I feel tired, but I must keep going; I have to make this journey. "You are not going anywhere," someone says.

"Why are you talking to me like this? My son will be here soon, and you will have to answer to him," I yell back.

"I am your son," this someone says.

You will never win an argument with a dementia patient. No matter their mental state, your loved ones are still the people you love; your parents are still your parents. You cannot distance yourself from the patient you are caring for, the same way that a professional caregiver is able to. When emotions are running high, change your reaction. It's extremely difficult to see tears

running down the face of your parent, especially when you compare the distraught person in front of you with how you remember your parent to be a few years ago: a column of strength and reassurance. Speak less, use fewer words, and rely on more body language to convey a message. The patient has diminished reasoning ability, and new techniques of communication are necessary.

A Son Coming to Grips with the Harsh Reality of Dementia

"You might be poor, your shoes might be broken, but your mind is a palace."
Frank McCourt

Our brother suffered terribly. As the man in the family, he felt the heavy burden of responsibility. But he remained stoic and never shared his frustrations. A few years after the initial diagnosis, he made a decision to share portions of his diary with us. I was so moved by his gesture that I made copies of some of his entries. For this book, I've picked the following three entries that poignantly describe his helplessness and the emotions he kept stoppered in a bottle that he couldn't uncap. These were made just before he got married, and just before he became a father, and he endured tremendous sadness that our mother couldn't be fully present for the joyous milestones in his life.

Entry #1

I cannot reason with you anymore; you don't seem to understand me when I speak to you. You are on a long journey. This journey, I am afraid, is forever. How can I stop you from wanting to walk out the door? What can I say that will make you understand me? How can I understand you and, more so, how can I help you?

Our lives have changed. The dynamics are no longer the same. You took care of me, and it is understandable that I now have to take care of you. Your sickness is hampering the natural progression of life, as you would have had so many more years of independence ahead of you. I have to take care of you now, to make sure you are safe. I'm finding it hard to accept the change in you. My friend, Ian, stopped by recently, and I told him of your dementia. He was surprised to hear this and did not know how to react. He tried to be empathetic, but I could sense some kind of awkwardness. I have to keep this to myself. I just can't let friends around me anymore, because they will think my family is crazy; or worse yet, they may be afraid that this is some kind of contagious disease.

I will be married soon, to a wonderful person who is compassionate and understanding. I am happy to have her in my life. Somehow, I cannot get my mother to remember her and recognize her as her future daughter-in-law. How can I get married and not let my mother know? I now have to watch helplessly as my mother goes on a lonely journey. It is the beginning of my long goodbye.

I wonder if there is a return. I wonder if I can do something, anything, to have my mother return from this mental confusion we are calling the journey. I pray that her return to normalcy will one day be made real. I go on my own mental trips, hoping that there is a cure for Alzheimer's, but it's just my imagination. I know, from my research and information from the doctor, that there is not yet a cure for this disease, and that I just have to watch my mom as she progresses from one diminished state to another, the latest one worse than the one before.

This journey will someday have a final destination. I know I have to cherish the moment and be lucky that I still have my mother. Sometimes it seems as though her degenerative condition is a mistake. I am excited at the little windows that open into normalcy—when I get a sensible reply to a question, a comment that flows from our conversation, or a gesture that seems familiar. I know that I have to move on with my life, knowing that my mother will not be there to support me as her journey unwinds.

I struggle to come to terms with this experience. This is the harsh reality. It is as if she has taken off on a jet plane and I am waving goodbye, but the plane stays grounded. Then a thought hits me. What if I ask an important question that she may recall the answer to? It is a struggle to find the sheerest glimmer of hope. It is as if I have one last dollar for a loaf of bread, but the bill is soaked and torn in my pocket. I know I have it, but I can't spend it. I have to listen to my mother's hallucinations all day. The total change of behaviour has made every interaction challenging. In the end, she is my mother, and I need to take control of myself to keep her safe. My sisters look to me for guidance, as we have to find new ways to cope with her condition.

Alzheimer's disease can be difficult to handle, especially if the patient exhibits many other symptoms of the disease, such as agitation, anxiety, and constantly wanting to escape. Caregivers experience firsthand the difficulties that this poses to both parties, the afflicted and the caregiver. Gain the confidence by maintaining self-control, and take steps to avoid getting stressed out, muddled, or exasperated.

A Memory of Better Times

"To understand something properly, we need to know it a little more;
but to know someone purely, we need to understand our inner feelings
truly and for sure."
Anuj Somany

Entry #2

My mother is not fond of strangers, so my future wife cannot be around her. She has to stay out of her sight. My mother is always accusing her of stealing her things—imaginary things. My fiancée is defenseless.

Her world is filled with contorted dimensions, distorted visions, and garbled communications. In her world, she is always right. No one can challenge her; there is no room for insubordination. I have to step up to the plate, to give her as much help as she needs. I am her only son, and I know she loves me and wants the best in the world for me. However, the way she expresses her love is tangled and is now often unspoken. It's not her fault. I am obedient and act as if things are normal. I know she can sense the difference in my behaviour; I see it from her reaction. She calls me all the time and grows increasingly agitated if I am not there to comfort her.

She loves my sisters, but in her confused state, her attachment to her son rings truest and clearest for me. We understand that she doesn't mean to express such a clear preference. Along with some limitations, we go along with what she wants. This is my mother's world now, and I have to stay connected with her to keep us all sane.

I am angry that you are this way, Mum. I am saddened that the mother we knew has disappeared before our eyes. We cannot reach you to recall good times or to have a good laugh about fun times from the past.

I remember that you would take me to school when I was young. You were always dressed up. You would join in our play and buy each of us ice-cream in the cafeteria. All my friends looked forward to seeing you at school. When I became a teenager, you were always there for me. I remember when I brought home my first girlfriend; the advice you gave me then, well, that will stay with me for the rest of my life.

What do I need to say or do or know now, before it becomes too late? There is no answer to be had, as it is already too late. I know you will not remember, but I will talk to you anyway. There may still be parts of your brain that have control of some senses. I will cherish you until you are no more. My life has changed and so has my family.

Entry #3

I am having your grandbaby. I know you may not recognize him, but I'll let you see and hold him. I am married now. We signed some papers in the chapel of the Catholic Church, just my wife and me and my sisters. It was at the church we would go to as a family. My wife still loves you and sends you all her affection and concern. I sometimes wonder why this happened to me, and why this happened to you, someone that I love and cherish.

I have to let go of this anger, and realize that things happen at random. Life is a hit and miss; sometimes there are good things, and then there are the not-so-good things. But I will not be mad at God for sending you on this journey. I will be grateful for the times you were there for us, and for the values that you instilled in me, which I will pass on to my little one. You have made me the man that I am today, and I will be ever grateful. When my son arrives, I will show you pictures, and I will tell him all about you. I will instill the same virtues in him that you did in me. I will read books, tell him stories, and sing him songs, and when he is older, I will go to his prom and dance at his prom night. You do not remember any of what you taught me, but your lessons will live, through me to him.

Do you want breakfast? I have prepared some ham and eggs and baked bread—your favorite. I am concerned about your health. I will do what I can to keep you safe, to keep you strong.

This disease has such a grip on the mind that individuals cannot express the way they feel. Even though they may be cognizant, there are changes taking place in them. It is important that caregivers have a firm grasp on the disease, and try their best to understand what the patient is feeling. The afflicted person does not need to be pitied, nor do you have to be endlessly melancholic around them. It is most crucial for their sense of well-being, or what's left of it, that they understand they are not alone. Whoever the caregiver might be, he or she must always be caring, considerate, and compassionate.

Keeping Connected

"I would not bend. They could not make me pliable.
My mind was strong. My mind was mine."
Janice Hardy

Some years went by, and our mother constantly repeated her urge to visit with her brother. It was like a broken record, with the needle stuck on the same tracks over and over again. As her kids, we gave her our undivided attention as much as we could, to not trigger a negative state of mind, which would last for days on end.

The Alzheimer's disease continued its unyielding march of devastation. We rallied around her, taking turns to provide continued supervision and care. Our mother was still a healthy woman in many ways, if we overlooked the fact that her brain was on a one-way track to ruin.

We never found it easy to reconcile that the woman before us was the one we grew up with. She was always so bright and so full of life, and loved to be involved in our lives, spending as much time as possible with us and her grandchildren. She was never tired of sharing incredible stories from her rich, long history. She was an attractive woman. Though she measured not more than five feet in her stockinged feet, she had a powerful presence.

Our six-foot tall brother towered over her, but she was always in control of disciplining him. She took great pride in her appearance, and loved handbags of all shapes and colours. It was our turn, as children, to repay the love, kindness, and compassion shown to us by this amazing woman. In time spent together, we encouraged her reflections on her life, wherever she was able to contribute. We talked about her past, something she was prone to drift into. She liked cooking—it was a hobby—and was always baking different types of cookies or stirring up a concoction that we loved and wanted more of.

We talked about great times but were careful not to push too far, for fear of triggering unexpected emotional breakdowns or eruptions. Reminiscing was therapeutic for us. We needed to maintain that connection, that bond that our mother worked very hard to nurture, through long years of loving discipline and care to instill precious values in us... Working at keeping the connection intact and open was not easy. It was the one thing we could share, so we worked hard at maintaining the bond.

The most powerful and positive action toward a person with dementia is to establish a harmonious connection with that person. Be deliberate and conscious in making that connection. In these moments of connection, will come joy, delight, and playfulness. Treating someone with respect means we appreciate that they have lived a wonderful and special life, which is worth getting to know. This means that, as caregivers, we need to be willing to take time to interact without judgement, but with appreciation. The person with dementia has an invisible antenna with which to pick up feelings that emanate from you. Make that person feel valued and treasured. This helps to create an emotionally safe place for them to land from the heights of confusion. Smile, or sometimes laugh, as you enter their world, attentively, respectfully, and with genuine loving care.

Chapter -2-

Plight of a Family

"The best thing about the future is that it comes one day at a time."
Abraham Lincoln

Our Lives Were Forever Changed

Our family was forever altered. We did the best we could and provided the necessary care and safety. We watched how the disease changed the life of Victoria, my mother, and how it impacted our lives as well.

There was a different turn of events each week, and each situation required that we make adjustments, for her and for our families. The grandchildren were getting older and were starting to question her behaviour. She could not recognize them, but she knew they were kids, and thus had to be kind to them. We explained to the children and, in their own way, they loved their grand-mother as best as they could. She had taken care of us, and we decided to carry the burden of having her with us, to reciprocate what she had done for us. We thought that having her at home with us, rather than at some long-term care facility, was a good thing we were doing for her. She would be able to see us all the time. It was not an easy decision, and we had to live with the consequences.

We were terrified at leaving the house, but we had to work. We had to run er-rands; we had to take our children to school. Fortunately, there was always someone to act as a caregiver until one of us returned. There were no cell phones, but we carried pagers. When the pager beeped, it was always something to do with Mom. Once, the pager buzzed with urgency. She had barricaded herself with my baby in the room, refusing access to the babysitter. I returned home as quickly as I could. When I turned up, Mom was adamant that the babysitter intended to take the baby away, and she had to go immediately. I calmed her down, managing to convince her that the baby was safe. I allowed the babysitter to leave and had to find someone else to take over the job. That was just one of many incidents that required we break away from our routines, to attend to her immediately.

We watched Mom travel alone on this wretched road of dementia. No one could predict how long her journey would last, but we knew that one day, she would arrive at her destination. We wished she could have lived out her natural years without the destructive hitchhiker in her brain, the one that goes by the name, Alzheimer's. This unravelling of her personality, of her faculties, was not the natural course of life; old age is. The behaviour she exhibited was strange to everyone—friends and even close relatives. None of them could fully comprehend the scope of the illness. Initially, we kept her from their sight and out of the public eye. But when we finally understood that she had no control over what she did, we decided to take her out with us whenever we could. To add complications to her life to spare the sensibilities of others was to complicate and worsen her quality of life much more than it was already. There were moments of spontaneity, when her old self shone through, and we relished those moments of connection. They were the ones that reminded us that she was still there—*our mom.*

You have to give back. Your parents made countless sacrifices for you, and now that Mom or Dad is stricken with this unreasonable condition called Alzheimer's, step up and do your part. They may not have been perfect, and your siblings may not be forthcoming in support. But you have to be different; you have to be there for them with empathy and love, as they were there for you.

The Denial

"As every divided kingdom falls, so every mind divided between many studies confounds and saps itself."
Leonardo da Vinci

We thought it would get easier after a few years, and that the pieces of the puzzle—how we coped, how we took care of my mom, and the changed relationships in the family—would fall into place. How naïve it was of my siblings and me. Alzheimer's is progressive and degenerative shrinkage of the brain. I should have realized that there was no turning back once the disease had sunk its claws deep into her. Perhaps in the very early stages, we could have found help to slow or retard its progression. My brother became the power of attorney for Mom's estate, and was also in charge of her care. He was her firstborn, and took charge as the dominant male figure, like our father would have done, had he still been alive.

My brother delegated to us what he wanted done, responsibilities that we willingly embraced. I finally arrived, after several years, to the point where I could call the disease by its own name, Alzheimer's. We had avoided doing so in the beginning, as Mom shied away from talking about illness, and avoided dealing with legal matters and finance. As a result of this experience, we learned to make all adequate preparations for our own children.

We were a lucky family, and fortunate to have a mother like her. Even though she had only the most basic schooling, she had the know-it-all and the wherewithal to raise her children well. We stuck together as a family, in happiness and in sickness. We loved each other, no matter the circumstances. We had moments of sibling rivalry, but these were few and far between. Even if I could call the disease by its name, I couldn't wrap my head around the reality that our mother was afflicted with the illness. I woke up every day thinking that this was not really happening, and that someday—yes, someday—it would all go away.

Feelings of hurt, conflict, sadness, and incredulity are inescapable. No matter how strong you think you are, you are vulnerable and bound to undergo anger, resentment, hate, love, and so on. These emotions, some very painful, are part of the process of dealing with a loved one with dementia. Bottling strong emotions and failing to express them is extremely damaging. There-fore, as the caregiver, you must go through a period of mourning. Spend some time expressing the way you feel, even if it means crying uncontrol-lably, laughing hysterically, or singing tunelessly out loud. When family members express emotions caused by grief, they bond. This is beautifully described by Paulo Coelho, in his book, The Alchemist. "When we love, we always strive to become better than we are. When we strive to become bet-ter than we are, everything around us becomes better too."

Outbursts and Eruptions

"And now these three remain: faith, hope and love.
But the greatest of these is love."
King James Version

I struggled to come to terms with this devastation called dementia. I wondered if there was something I needed to know, before the source of information shut down completely. My mother was always a fountain of information; she knew dates, times, and places. Without batting an eyelash, the answers were always ready at the tip of her tongue. The total change of behaviour had given rise to challenging situations, some beyond our control. This was our mother. We had to be as understanding as we were humanly capable of. She would swing from emotion to emotion, and erupted into anger without provocation or reason. That meant we had to be on watch all the time.

She had no intention of hurting us or the grandchildren, but if we let our atten-tion slip, she would find a way to inflict harm on herself. Once, we slipped some medication into her meal to keep her calm for a few days. Then, inexpli-cably, without cause, we heard a loud crash. She had thrown a kitchen pot through the glass window. We didn't understand the cause of her frustration, but it was clear to us that the sedation was wearing off. Although she was ex-hibiting the symptoms typical of sun-downing or restlessness in the late evening, a symptom common to Alzheimer's patients, we were not yet near dusk. The sun was bright overhead, and I realized that her latest outburst was the demon of the illness acting up in mid-day.

At some point, giving up control of the situation becomes necessary in order to yield the patient to more capable hands, such as professionals. You can't do it all, no matter how supportive your surrounding relationships may be. You are going to need all the help you can get. It's incredibly difficult and frustrating taking care of someone with Alzheimer's. This can be a long-term care facility of your choice. When you finally have that burden of care lifted off your shoulders, it is inevitable that you would wish you had done it earlier. Seeking professional long-term care is an action to take for the well-being of the patient, and for you, the caregiver, and the rest of the family.

Anger, Frustration, and Guilt

"Sometimes I ask myself, 'Do I have the courage to do the right thing when it matters most?'
And that answer, I'm afraid, is silence."
Jarod Kintz

Mary Tyler Moore once said, "You can't be brave if you've only had wonderful things happen to you." After coming to terms with my mother's condition, I understood those words better. I also better understood the disease. It was not easy to accept that this dreadful disease had invaded our home. However, it did make me stronger and brought our family closer together. I was not spared the emotions of anger, frustration, and guilt. I was angry to see my mother struck before her time, furious to witness her deterioration with my own eyes, and frustrated that I could only watch helplessly. I became angry when she forgot our names, because for her to lose the maternal instinct was to me the final straw.

I shuddered with frustration when I saw how her hallucinations affected all of us. Her confusion and her delusions were intangible. What she was going through was happening in the shadowy realms of her mind. I felt guilty when we locked the doors to the house, and the front and back gates. Each time we left, we were in a mild state of panic for fear that we would, on our return, find her whole and in full possession of her faculties. If so, deliberately locking her in the house would have been a tragic and sad mistake.

The grandchildren, the next generation, were only able to talk to the physical vessel that was once occupied by a warm and loving person. We were happy and grateful to have her with us, but we were always angry that she was not more fully present. We were tasked with learning about the disease, once we figured what it was, and we learned quickly. I was always riddled with the fear that we should be doing more. I was often afraid that we might one day give up or give in to our frustration. I felt guilty that we had not acted sooner. Had we done so, maybe we would have had more time to prepare for the manifestation of the disease and the onslaught of irrational behavior, memory loss, and hallucinations. We ignored her early complaints of a failing memory. After all, she had always been as sharp as a tack recalling the smallest and most inconsequential detail for as long as I could remember. Maybe it was our fault that she became ill.

At times, as her caregiver, her overbearing behaviour felt frustrating. But in the next moment, I would be struck with the guilt of being impatient with her. During the calm and rewarding days, we were able to exchange ideas, and enjoyed each other's company. Yet how could I be happy when someone that I loved was no longer themselves? I felt sad that she could not be part of my happiness that I had presently and that I would have in the future. Instead, I was part of her decline to her demise. Even though I harbored tremendous guilt, that emotion also catalyzed me into action. However, it was in compassion that I found my strength to view the situation as objectively as I could, and it was from compassion that I chose to always act in good faith.

Caregivers often suffer guilt. That emotion should have no place in the relationship between the caregiver and the loved one, but guilt is the hardest emotion to extricate. Watching your loved one increasingly degenerate, while you remain strong and healthy, can tear you apart if you give in to the guilt. Try instead to release the feelings of guilt, and focus on the task at hand of being a caretaker to someone who needs your complete attention. The time will come when you will have to make the painful decision to enrol your loved one in a long-term care facility. Use your interim time wisely to consult with other members of the family, family doctors, and other caretakers so that, when the moment comes to make the move, it is less painful for all involved. If coping is really difficult, speaking to a counsellor can help significantly.

Chapter -3-

How Prepared Are We To Look at Death as a Reality?

"I am not sure exactly what heaven will be like, but I know that when we die and it comes time for God to judge us, he will not ask, 'How many good things have you done in your life?' Rather, he will ask, 'How much love did you put into what you did."
Mother Teresa

The Deafening Calm

The nightly rituals of pacing, talking, and shouting to invisible strangers continued. Once in a long while, she would go to bed and have a normal sleep without medication. It wasn't always easy to slip the pills into her food or drink. She was always on the go, always wanting to do something, whether it was a meaningful act or not. After a few years, Alzheimer's had fully taken residence in my mother's brain. Although she still walked, her movements were not as strong as in the earlier years.

We were always conscious of making the physical environment safe for her, and there was always constant supervision. The intelligible noises she made became part of our lives. Our ears and minds became familiar with the sounds of her confusion. One day, as if by magic, the noises went away. It was quiet. It felt like the calm before the storm broke—the silence felt abnormal; it was not kind. She no longer laughed, nor did she high-five her grandchildren.

This sudden turn of events had us all confused. I wondered how this could be possible; she was doing fine in her world and, suddenly, this deafening silence descended on us. We watched her sitting, or at rest, in utter quiet. I thought we were being tested again, as I recalled the saying, "When it's your time, it's your time." Nothing we did previously prepared us for the inevitable. I knew that one day the "big rest" would claim her, as it would all of us in the natural ebb and flow of life. We died when we got old, to make room for the young children that came after us.

The day began as it normally did, in the most routine way. The caregiver walked into the house, and I headed off to work. I was at work, and my siblings were on and about their day's errands. I was just settling in my office when my pager went off. This was not unusual, and as I picked up the phone, I asked myself, "What now?"

The caregiver was frantic on the other end of the line. My mother was in trouble. Even though I asked what had happened, I decided not to wait for the full explanation because, every second I was on the phone, something else could happen. I hung up abruptly, quickly found my boss, and asked for permission to leave as something had happened to my mother. I was in a state of panic. This was an entirely different call, and I was anxious. When I got home, no one was there. A neighbour called out to me, "Your mom is at the hospital; she got hit by a car."

My turbulent anxiety turned into cold fear. All I could ask was, "What hospital?" I next said, "Okay, I will find it," and hurried off without waiting for more information. I arrived at the hospital, and there was my mom, silent—the first time in a long time that she was saying nothing. She had been wounded, but the prognosis was okay. But I knew that, while she would recover from the physical injury, the mental wounds would never heal. I took a few weeks off work to care for my mother. She was never the same after the fortnight's stay in the hospital. We could not blame the caregiver for leaving the gate unlocked, we could not judge the guilty party, nor could we continue to anguish in what should have been.

There was a new task facing us. Mom stayed in bed most of the time after this incident. We got her up from time to time, but it was too much for her. The quietness in the house deafened us. We missed the noise and the uproar; at least then we knew that she was alert, even if the connections were jumbled. Now the opposite had arrived. After two years of battling an agonizing recovery, her time had arrived. It was her time to find peace.

Our mother walked out of a seemingly secure environment into the path of a vehicle. We had tried to keep her as safe as possible, but our arrangements proved insufficient. She never recovered from that accident, and her physical body deteriorated. It was a struggle for us, as children, to accept that we had done the best we could with the information we were given at the time. She was only sixty-one when she left us, in a manner of speaking, and started her journey through her disease. Throughout so much of her illness, we did not understand and could not make any sense of what was happening to her and to us. Though we knew nothing of Alzheimer's, and there was little information to be had at that time, we cherished and loved her anyway.

Accidents occur no matter how much you prepare for safety. Patients constantly seeking a way out—exit seekers—are the most vulnerable. Falls are also common. It is impossible to keep an eye on the patient all the time when there are other things that need to be done. There are now regulations in place for restraints such as seat belts and bed rails, which have been brought about by the number of accidental deaths. Support groups are great in sharing coping strategies and in offering emotional reinforcements.

A Portrayal

"It's so much darker when a light goes out
than it would have been if it had never shone."
John Steinbeck

The story above is the story of my mother, Victoria. This story started before her memory and cognitive ability continued its irreparable decline. Her journey into the abyss began long before she decided to visit her brother, a long trip that she could only complete in her mind. As I now reminisce on the old memories, I can't help but recall those times I saw her in the garden, her cigarette between her lips, one hand holding the container for the beans, and harvesting with the other. She could balance all three steps with precision and dexterity, smoking, holding, and picking. I often admired her. It seemed at these moments she found focused concentration. She found solace. It felt good for her to be released of old tensions as she touched the blooming trees, collected the vegetables, or swiped away the stubborn grasses that showed up sporadically. There was always something else to do as she pondered and lingered on. I watched those puffs of clouds float by, wishing that all these timeless treasures of the flow and warmth of her garden would bring her good health and happiness.

The beans she reaped would be for lunch or dinner, whichever time caught up with her. The garden was her place for tranquillity as it was scattered with towering fruit trees, and the vegetables she planted. The tropical blue sky, with white fluffy clouds floating in space, would often appear on the days she decided to wander through her garden for that pursuit of solitude. There was always noise everywhere, from the chickens, ducks, and other livestock she reared. She would cook her produce with great affection, even though there were no particular concepts to what was prepared. She had a knack for her concoctions. It tasted great, and we always wanted more.

My mother was a strong woman, and she had worked most of her life to support her family. She ironed clothes and sewed, cooked, cleaned, and grew the food we ate from her garden. She sold some of her vegetables and livestock to neighbours or passers-by for extra money. She took pride in her produce. It was also a way to connect with people as it was often the source of her conversation. She had an unerring ability to understand the conditions that could lead to a good crop. She, however, wasn't good in business. If the customer came to her with a story of hardship, my mother would give the vegetables away for a pittance. She often stood at the kitchen window, a cigarette in one hand and a cup of coffee in the other. She would stand looking over her garden, admiring her crops. At intervals, she would place the cup on the countertop while she took a puff of her cigarette.

She chain smoked, a habit she adapted from very young. Beneath the canopy of her peppered life, as a child, and having her own children to care for, she was certain not to duplicate her past or repeat the present. Her motivation for life was strong. She willed herself to be inspired by her own daunting childhood, to raise her own children with dignity. My brother towered over my mother, but it did not stop her from letting him know that smoking was forbidden. This was the one vice that was off limits and offensive for her children.

He would stand in front of her, humbled and bemused by this petite lady. She would occasionally say to him, "Smoking would not make you a man. Ever since you were a little boy, the things you've said and done have made me mad and made me proud. So as you get older, you cannot depart from my teaching. You will one day be the man of this house. Stop your foolish antics and be strong like your father." His emotions could not be visible. After all, he was on his way to manhood. Today, none of us have ever smoked a cigarette or any other kind of device.

Her deep spirituality was truly the gift that brought inner calm and peace in real life, with all its difficulties and problems surrounding her. Her inward journey was to love. Her focus was to bring happiness to her family and others. Her sense of humor was the quality that attracted others to her. Relatives or friends, strangers or neighbours, she made everyone feel as if they were best buddies, even on first meeting. She was extremely hospitable and always offered guests food. Often, she would walk over to her garden, pick up some vegetables, snatch up a chicken, and give it to a friend or even a stranger, with the admonition, "Go home and cook for your children." In the art of her giving, she gained incredible satisfaction and gratefulness for what she received.

Helping others made her happy; smiles and laughter filled our humble home. She was fun to have around. As adults, we still looked to her for advice and guidance; she had a lot of wisdom to give for a woman with meagre schooling. Her advice was impeccable, her confidence was admirable, and she was fearless. She solved every problem with the same bold confidence.

For example, on occasion, she would walk over to talk to Fred, after she caught wind that he had a fight with his "children's mother," his common-law wife. Try as we might have, we could not talk her out of interfering, because her motherly instinct was to restore peace. Often, she would help settle a tiff or sort out a squabble. However, when it came to her turn, the problem was bigger than she could handle; it was larger than her experience afforded her, and there was nothing she could do. Alzheimer's caught her in an escapable grip from which she couldn't escape, strong as she was. It kept its inexorable hold on her mind, and weakened its opponent to submission, while all the time preparing the ring for the eventual and inevitable knockout.

The Final Separation

*"There are moments when I wish I could roll back the clock
and take all the sadness away, but I have the feeling that if I did,
the joy would be gone as well."*
Nicholas Sparks

On a warm Friday afternoon in January, I stood by my mother's bedside, watching her final separation. January was the month she entered this world, and the month she would exit. I listened to the words of her favorite song as it played softly in the background. It was "Amazing Grace." The words of this song touched me deeply as I thought how fitting the ambiance was for a life well lived. The lyrics expressed this sentiment in a profound way, reflective of her simple life, but rich with the innate ethical qualities of a mom: *"Yea, when this flesh and heart shall fail, and mortal life shall cease, I shall profess, within the vale, a life of joy and peace. The earth shall soon dissolve like snow, the sun forbear to shine; but God, who called me here below, will be forever mine."* She sang and hummed this song often while she cooked and cleaned the house. It was sung often with humility at a local Baptist church she attended at times.

This is a song of gratitude, and my mother had a lot to be grateful for. Her hard life as a child, and the difficulty with her husband's shortcomings, and his eventual death, shaped her every moment. She was giving, pleasant, and strict with us as her children. She, in her wisdom, arising from her challenges of pain and sufferings, wanted us not to repeat her pattern of life. She was always thanking God for something accomplished, or offering what little she had to anyone who she thought needed a little help, as she always humbly uttered. It was her way of looking out for others and making them happy. This was her final day for judgment. All that she was, and all that she could have been, was summed up at that moment. We, the jurors, deliberated long and hard, and still no affirm verdict for a cure of the disease that took the life of Victoria.

In nursing, I have had many opportunities to watch other families go through the final separation, which takes the loved one away from them forever. It seemed my mother had traveled a long and tiring road. This final destination was, for us as bystanders, bittersweet. The memory of her bubbly personality, her infectious laughter, and the compendium of knowledge from her college of hard knocks, will forever be etched in our memories.

One thing is for sure. If you loved them enough, theirs would have been a life of joy. This thought gave us, family and caregivers hope that there was peace at the end of this last and final step she had to take. We had no control over the timing or hour of death, and even though it was expected, the final hour still descended suddenly. There was a sense of unreality when it happened. There was a cacophony of emotions. Was it really taking place, this inevitable and final separation? Was I really witnessing my mother's departure? I was irked that I no longer had a routine around my mom, to bathe, feed, and clothe her. Her being gone was the harsh reality and, once again, my life was forever altered.

A question was asked: "What is dying?" And the answer returned, "Her diminished size and loss of sight is in me, not in her." And just at the moment when someone at my side says, "She is gone," there are others who are watching her coming, gladly shouting, "Here she comes!" And that is dying. This perception of dying for someone you loved grappled for my comprehension.

Rather than anxiety or apprehension among us, we felt nothing but love, infused with the understanding that "rest" for our mother meant being in the gentle embrace of angelic hosts. Just knowing her life story, experiences, circumstances, and eventual sorrows, changed my understanding of these emotional dynamics to a response of compassion.

I realized that death is not to be feared, because it is not the end but a passage to eternity. The peace and calm just before death signifies that suffering disappears in the physical. At this juncture, I thought of the unspoken dialogue that we carry around all the time—the questions we could have asked, the songs we could have sang, and the value we could have experienced, appreciating more of what she felt—and I wondered what Mom's was, nearing the end of her journey.

The Departure

*"The boundaries which divide life from death
are at best shadowy and vague.
Who shall say where one ends and the other begins?"*
Edgar Alan Poe

You prepared us well in advance of this impending outcome. We had the time to grieve your loss when you disappeared before our eyes. We watched you as you sank slowly into the dark abyss. We saw the separation between your personality and the body that contained our mother. The memories that cemented the bonds between us, with relatives and friends, were the first to go. Your character traits that made you special, and your infectious laughter and warm heart were the next to depart, winging into a distant place we could not reach, and we could no longer share fun memories. And when you slipped in and out of consciousness in the final stages, we were relieved to know that you were nearing your final destination.

We have held you, loved you, and watched over you, and now we must let you go. Amidst the soft music of "Amazing Grace" in the background, a song that you loved, tranquility came over you. It was the calm to herald you into another dimension, the one we called heaven. We were prepared; we had shed our tears, and we had a long time to say goodbye.

That is the difference between Alzheimer's disease and other illnesses. There is a slow death of the personality and of the mind, and it begins many years before the ending of the physical body.

A Farewell

"Life has to end," she said. "Love doesn't."
Mitch Albom

As I stood there among the many mourners, who were dressed in their sombre blacks and whites, I thought it fitting that a woman, who had lived her life not only for her family, but who also gave of herself to anyone who came in contact with her, would have many coming to pay their final respects and to say farewell. She was unselfish in the way she helped and gave. She was always happy, evoking laughter with her unique sense of humor, and spicing up life with her creative ideas. This was a blessed day, I thought to myself on this bright sunny day. My mother had found freedom; she was at last free of the merciless clench of Alzheimer's disease. I felt that all who were gathered there that day shared my sentiments. It was a good day to revisit the happy times and the not-so-happy times. There was food and drinks after we laid her to rest. I returned to the home in which she had spent many, many years in a better frame of mind.

I would be forever grateful for her existence and the many lessons her journey had taught me. My mother would be pleased to know that the time she invested in training and bringing up her family yielded the dividend she always expected. She taught us to do good, to help others, and to instill those solid values in our own families.

Expressing Appreciation

"At the end of the day, let there be no excuses,
no explanations, no regrets."
Steve Maraboli

The ravages of this dreaded disease, Alzheimer's, took its victim on a relentless quest to her final destination, while all the time destroying the fibres of her existence and of her mind. She never recalled the start of the journey, and she never knew when she arrived. Her mind just simply wouldn't let her process. She failed to recognize her children at some point, but she understood the universal language of love. No matter how jumbled her thoughts were, she knew that she was loved. She may never have understood it when we told her that she was the best mom. We often did, but she failed to respond. She couldn't.

When we said we were sorry, she could not appease us by saying," It's not your fault." She would never know that we cared. The frustrations that we felt, and the efforts to keep her safe and calm, did not always produce our hoped-for results. However, we knew that even if she couldn't express or respond in kind, she could feel it.

It was as if the cycle of life had reversed itself. From her role as an adult, it appeared that time unwound, and she became more and more childlike. It was not her fault that she wanted to go on a journey that never was, to seek for things that were not there, and to chase away people that only her confused mind could see. We, the families, could only hop on the unwanted ride. It was not a journey we would have willingly joined, if given the choice.

There are families around the world who have survived this painful journey, and there are families who are just starting out. I will say that families that endure, remain steadfast, and stick together throughout this torturous journey, bear an indelible mark of courage. The love and care that caregivers, families, and professional caretakers give unselfishly, is to be commended. These are the unsung heroes.

There are countless other diseases and illnesses that require time and patience on the part of the families. The weight they bear is equally as heavy. At this point, I salute the caregivers, and I say, "Thank you for a job well done." I say this on behalf of the victims, including my mother. Had she been alive today, and were it before illness cut her in her prime, she would most certainly find a trinket in her cupboard to reward you for your long and untiring work to keep company with those who have to travel this unexpected and painful journey.

Chapter -4-

The Stigma

"Nobody cares how much you know,
until they know how much they care."
Theodore Roosevelt

Amidst all the events of my life, I found myself in the field of nursing. This was a special calling; it was righteous energy, and it was my mother who suffered from the effects of Alzheimer's disease. It had been quite a while since I had been among a network of friends and associates, and at no time did I ever speak of my mother's demise. My emotional sensitivity was still too fresh to repeat the details of her traumatic events, and most of all, the stigma. The stigma attached to having Alzheimer's was too disconcerting to perceive.

As I continued to do my job, with a fierce determination to do my best, it was clear that I was there for a reason. I could say that my job was to take care of the necessities of daily life—food, clothes, shelter—but it was more. I began to take notice of the commonality among the patients I cared for. They all had families that loved them very much, and the empathy and compassion from which other nurses operated was too much to ignore. And most of these patients were affected by the disease of Alzheimer's and dementia.

My personal dignity, and love for others, fervently dominated my wakening hours. I began to love my job and look forward to another day with my patients. I had reasons to feel the love, empathy, and compassion. I had a secret; my mother had Alzheimer's. And so, when I touched a patient or gave an embrace, it reminded me of my mother. The burden of guilt from not knowing enough of her condition was continually pursuing me.

I was visiting at a bank one Tuesday morning and sat with a financial planner. She knew me from my frequent visits and as an avid customer with that branch of the bank. As we began to speak, she made eye contact with a well-dressed gentleman as he entered the bank and took his position in the already formed line, leading toward the tellers. She looked at him from the corner of her eye, from her small cubicle. As he procured his full position in the line, and was now in full view, she stared a little longer at him. I wondered for a while what the fascination was; he looked normal, was well-groomed, and had a definite purpose. There was a pause, then the reveal. She turned to me and whispered, "See that man? He has Alzheimer's. He comes to the bank and does not know what he is here to do. We have to call his family to come and get him."

I kept silent for a few seconds as I searched my thoughts for a reply. I knew the bank clerk only said this to me because she knew I worked with Alzheimer's and dementia patients. I broke my silence; I had to respond. I could only talk from my experience. I could think only of my mother, as I took a firm look at the well-dressed man. It was then that the words came, and for the first time, I uttered, "My mother had Alzheimer's." As I said those words, tears rimmed my eyes as though I was seeing her through the lens of his eyes. It was then that I began to tell her of my escapade with my mother. She was ready and anxious to hear, and with a genuine desire, she listened. It was just a synopsis. I took a few minutes, but it seemed like an hour; after all, we had jobs to do. However, I felt inspired and progressive. I felt reprieved; I felt free.

I left the bank, not only with what I was there to accomplish, but with a personal transformation. My self-confidence was tremendous. I can now do anything; I can write my book. As I continued to drive home, I proclaimed, "I will tell the world about my mother. I will not hide the fact that she had Alzheimer's. I can share my story with other families going through their own journeys." The experience with my mother, and the fact that I work at a long-term care facility, gave me firsthand knowledge of this disease, enough to share, as I care very much about the changes that it brings to families. My passion to write, and my love, compassion and courage as a caregiver, gave me the substance. I just needed the connection.

This disease has such a grip on the mind that individuals cannot express the way they feel. Even though they may be cognizant, there are changes taking place in them. It is important that caregivers have a firm grasp on the disease and try their best to understand what the patient is feeling. It is most crucial for their sense of well-being, or what's left of it, that they understand they are not alone. Whoever the caregiver might be, he or she must always be caring, considerate, and compassionate.

I often wonder what it would be like if my mother could have expressed the way she felt. As I go through my daily routine at my place of employment, I draw my own conclusion from the patients I work with. Though Alzheimer's and dementia steal the very essence of one's existence, there is always that window of coherence or self-expression. I know she would have left us a message before embarking on her journey. Through my experience, and to put into perspective the nature of the disease, it would have sounded like this.

My children,

I have four of you, but I dare not tell which one of you will take care of me, as I take care of you. This choice is for you and your family to decide. However, as I envision my future, I can only imagine what I would like it to be. So as I appeal to your better judgement, I ask that you take me in and be patient with me. Please understand that my memory is not what it is used to be. I forget things a lot, which will frustrate and upset you. Understand what I am going through. I am irritated and confused but cannot express it in words that hold true for you. I may forget what I say in minutes, but I will remember how you made me feel.

Understand that I will repeat myself many times; I will ask that same question several times. I ask that you go along, and know that this is my new normal. Know that my condition will not get better, so have an open heart and judge me on what I once was. Please remember those times, and honor me in the caring for which I am preparing you.

As my condition of Alzheimer's progresses, which is the truth that I could not face, it will arrive in its glory, and take over my cognitive abilities. There will be times when I will not want to do the thing you want me to. I will be very defiant at times, but know that this is all part of the process, and that I have no control of my actions. Just be patient with me. I want you to know that I want to be with you, and that sending me away, because you cannot cope, will only depress me and make me agitated.

You are my children, and I took care of you, and each of you turned out very well. I am a proud parent. It's your turn to be with your own families, and I surely would not interfere with your family routine. However, I am not looking for you to reciprocate, because I believe it was my duty to raise healthy and respectful children. I am looking forward to your compassion and love. With a little empathy, find the courage to accept me in my circumstance. As I get older, and with my diminished reasoning abilities, please find the time to accept me in your daily routine until it's time for me to enter the eternal kingdom.

I love you.

The Grieving Process

"Grief is not a disorder, a disease or a sign of weakness.
It is an emotional, physical and spiritual necessity,
and the price you pay for love. The only cure for grief is to grieve."
Earl Crollman

The grieving process occurs after the loved one's final passing. However, if you are in the phase of anticipatory grief, you may experience some or even all of the five stages of grief during this time. It will be beneficial for you to read through this section to better handle your emotional turbulence. This will ultimately help you help others who are also grieving.

No one can tell you exactly how to heal. You may decide to ask others for help and hope, and you absolutely should. However, if you are constantly depending upon others rather than your own intuition and insight, you could be led astray, or take a long time to heal. Everyone must undergo their own individual experience when it comes to grieving. Receive plenty of comfort, accept the pain as it comes, and give out hugs.

From the beginning stages of caregiving for someone with Alzheimer's, to the very end, your heart—your emotional centre—undergoes a lot of stress and despair. For those of you who have not previously encountered death, the pain of loss can be extremely cutting. Even if you have grieved ahead of time, the actual occurrence of death will be shocking to your soul.

Sometimes a survivor copes with the shock by indulging in denial, which is the first stage of grief. Another may suffer survivor's guilt, which is guilt that you are still alive and able to fully experience and enjoy this world. Survivor's guilt is known to bring about severe loneliness and isolation. If you must, allow yourself to experience these emotions. Just don't forget to move forward to reality. Your loved one is not angry that you are still alive, and you can best honor his or her memory by living your own life fully.

Everyone grieves in his or her own way and time. But the longer you push the pain away, the worse it becomes. Pain never just dissipates. It must be felt and fully accepted in order to leave at some point in the future. Pain that is repressed gets lodged in the body. Many people get sick and even become diagnosed with potentially deadly diseases during times of grief. This isn't true just for those who push pain away. This is also true for those who become overwhelmed with too much sorrow and emotional pain.

It's important to have some balance during the grieving process. Seek out inspiration, hope, and healing in every way that you can. Staying away from family members and friends can also be extremely harmful.

If you are having a difficult time finding appropriate balance between grieving and living your life, find a counselor. Many grief counselors also provide group therapy, but you can also find additional group therapy elsewhere; some churches provide group sessions that are focused on the pain of grief. Either way, dealing with your pain is the most healing thing you can do for your own soul.

The Five Stages of Grief

There are five stages of grief, but not everyone experiences each stage. Ignoring your feelings, or *DENIAL*, is the first stage of grief. This is normal, but it is also classified, under popular psychology, as a defense mechanism. Denial acts as an insulating cushion during the initial shock. You may isolate yourself, and that's fine as long as it's temporary. Hopefully, you will move forward in the grieving process.

The second stage of grief is *ANGER*. You have every right to be angry; it is not wrong as long as you don't cause harm to others when you release it. Anger stems from many sources, including feeling helplessness, fear, and confusion. Don't let it get the better of you. Instead, be aware of why you are angry and, with that consciousness, find a way to defuse it.

You become angry because you don't want to own this awful pain of loss. Some people get angry at God or even rail at their loved ones who are no longer with them. If you get to this stage of grieving and begin to feel guilty because of your anger, know that you are not alone.

The third stage of grieving is known as *BARGAINING*. This stage is more likely to occur during anticipatory grief. Every stage of grief that I am describing can occur during both anticipatory and actual grief. Bargaining comes from the need to control life. You might attempt to make deals with God to postpone your loved one's death.

Some may beat themself up with accusations against themselves, with such statements as, "If only I was more loving," or "If only I kept them alive longer." Since you cannot change what has already happened, it isn't advisable to pour more guilt upon yourself. However, these feelings are perfectly normal, so let them all out. Be completely honest with how you feel, and accept your emotions as true, real, and healthy.

DEPRESSION is the fourth stage of grief, and it can last a long time. You first feel grief and sorrow when you realize that you won't see your loved one again. Depression occurs when you settle in to life without them, and you realize how sad that can be. You greatly miss your loved one and aren't sure how to go on with life. It's going to take time to learn a new way of living. Nothing will ever be the same again, and this truth is the most difficult thing to accept.

ACCEPTANCE is the fifth and final stage of grief. It may take months or even years to get to this point. Acceptance is felt in a variety of ways. You may start crying more than you did at first or you may stop crying altogether. Some people come to terms with everything at the beginning of the grieving process, but this acceptance has not yet taken up full residency in the heart.

No matter what stage of grief you are in, do your best to allow your heart to accept the pain as it comes. No one wants to feel the pain of grief, but it's truly the only way to heal. It's natural to experience pain and suffering in life, and it should help you to know that you aren't alone. Take as much love as is given to you. Above all, love yourself as much as possible. It's not going to be easy, but it will be worth it.

Getting Back to Life

"Someday you're going to look back on this moment
of your life as such a sweet time of grieving.
You'll see that you were in mourning
and your heart was broken, but your life was changing."
Elizabeth Gilbert

Life after the death of a loved one is different, and you must accept that. Moving forward is the hardest thing to do, even if you have reached the final stage of grief. Sorrow paralyzes the soul, the mind, the will, and the heart. Your slump into apathy can easily consume you, and you won't feel like doing anything.

The first way to conquer this apathy and excessive sorrow is to change your thoughts. Changing how and what you think is the simplest action you can take, although it is not easy by any means. For example, if you keep telling yourself things like, "I just can't move on," or "I cannot live my life without him or her," it's almost guaranteed that you won't move on or live your life. We don't realize how powerful we are until we are forced to access the power of our own minds.

Instead of believing the lie that you cannot move on, tell yourself something else that is comforting and empowering. Say out loud to yourself, "I can begin moving forward little by little, and eventually I will be able to enjoy life." Say, "I can eventually live a brand new life, and it may feel awkward at first, but I will get used to it."

Speaking out loud is a very powerful, therapeutic tool that will inspire you and bring healing. There are millions of potential statements that you can speak out loud, so make sure to say them as much as needed until your heart truly believes them.

Once you believe the truth in your words, you will have the willpower to act upon it. Healing takes time, and no one heals in the exact same way, but there are tools available to help you in the process. When you begin to feel your emotions and inner strength building up, this is when you will be able to take action.

Real healing is found in action. After grief, often comes fear. Fear might isolate you from other people, or it might make you clingy and needy. Don't let this fear take over. Rise up and take a stand, using all the courage that you can muster.

Creating new memories will help to replace the old ones, and new memories will bring joy and peace to a suffering soul. You may not necessarily subscribe to this as you are experiencing new ways of living, but as you look back to these new memories, you will see that this is true.

At this point, you may be wondering what actions you can take. At the very start, don't place overwhelming expectations upon yourself. Do things that are easy. Get together with friends and family for an outing and a dinner.

Now that you have experienced the mourning of a lost loved one, you may never look at life the same way. This is a good thing. You can become stronger and more passionate about life than you ever were before.

If you are reading this book before experiencing the passing and mourning of a loved one, create a plan of action ahead of time. When you finally come to the place of mourning, you may not have the ability to think clearly. Even if you become a little bit stronger each day, such details may be overwhelming when you are emotionally delicate and vulnerable. Pre-planning and writing out a list of things that you can do, places you can travel to, and people you can spend time with, may make it easier for you to follow through with action.

Activities that bring you closer to your lost loved one may prove to be healing. Listen to your loved one's favorite songs, watch their favorite television shows and movies, and read their much loved books. You can even visit some of their preferred places or cook their favorite meals. While it is important that your life not become a shrine to theirs, there is nothing wrong with keeping them close to you.

Celebrate Their Life!

"Lost love is still love, Eddie. It just takes a different form, that's all.
You can't hold their hand...You can't tousle their hair...
But when those senses weaken, another one comes to life...
Memory...Memory becomes your partner.
You hold it...you dance with it...Life has to end,
Eddie...Love doesn't."
Mitch Albom

While keeping your lost loved one close to you is healthy, focusing more upon them than on your own existence is extremely unhealthy. You are depending upon someone who is now only available in spirit. Instead of attempting to get love from them, give it back to them, by celebrating the life they lived. This will not only heal your heart, but it will bring fulfillment to your life.

It's widely known by many who have grieved before you that celebrating the life of the one who has gone helps you heal much faster. Everyone does this differently, but the feelings of joy, hope, and peace are the same. We all need inner healing, whether or not we have experienced loss. Joy is desirable to healing, and it is the other face of sadness. Whatever you can do to create this joy and happiness will revive you from the depths of despair.

Besides reminiscing with friends and family, you can decide to create a scrapbook of your lost loved one. Find special items to include in this scrapbook ahead of time. Take lots of pictures, and gather old ones that have been stored away in photo albums. Gather some pictures of their favorite things and, if you can, try to collect things that would actually fit in the scrapbook ahead of time.

Creating new memories helps to heal the heart, because creating memories is the essence of life; it is the core of living. It's not the memories themselves that are important. Instead, it's the sensory, emotional, and physical experience, and the contentment and satisfaction that arises from living fully, that gives birth to precious memories.

Concentrate on yourself. Remember your loved one. Try your best not to make excuses to avoid life. Your loved one wants you to live life to the fullest. Honor them by doing just that! Ultimately, celebrate their life by reveling in the joy of your own.

Chapter -5-

Dementia And the Brain

"Alzheimer's is the cleverest thief, because she not only steals from you, but she steals the very thing you need to remember what's been stolen."
Jarod Kintz

What Is Dementia?

Dementia refers to a clinical disorder and describes a group of symptoms that severely affect and interfere with thinking and social functions. Dementia is not a disease, but rather a disorder that can be associated with many different underlying diseases. Dementia impairment of cognitive function is widespread. It can involve different combinations of impaired brain functions, affecting memory for events, and the understanding of facts, language, thinking, and reasoning, and even the perception of the world. It is also characterized by disorientation and difficulties with decision-making that affect daily life.

Alzheimer's is the most common cause of dementia. The other degenerative diseases that lead to dementia affect different areas of the cerebral cortex. Since different parts of the cortex specialize in different body functions, the disease will manifest in deficiency of the function that is affected, such as having problems with lucidity, or problems with language or body movements. There are many types of dementia, each with its own features that separate one from another.

Types of Dementia

Alzheimer's Disease Dementia

Alzheimer's disease is a long, slow, progressive mental and physical deterioration of the brain. The name *Alzheimer's disease* came from the renowned researcher, pathologist, and neurologist, Alois Alzheimer, who was of German decent. In 1906, Dr. Alzheimer studied parts of the brain of a fifty-seven-year-old woman who was struck by dementia. On her death, he analyzed sections of her brain. He observed what he called amyloid plaque (clumps of protein in the cortex and the hippocampus), neurofibrillary tangles (densely twisted bundles of fibrils, which are very fine fibres), and loss of nerve connections. He devoted a great deal of his scientific research to the mechanism by which the brain produces amyloid (abnormal protein), which degrades the neurons in the brain. Subsequent research into Alzheimer's disease shows atrophy (shrinkage); loss of brain cells; loss of brain chemicals, or neurotransmitters, that send signals from one part of the brain to the other; loss of cellular self-maintenance abilities; and persistent inflammation.

Alzheimer's is a chronic disease, and the first warning sign is abnormal memory impairment. As the disease advances, patients are unable to care for themselves, and the loss of brain function eventually leads to the failure of other systems in the body. This eventually leads to death, but usually only many years after the disease first takes its toll. Alzheimer's disease has emerged as one of the most common brain disorders. It is the dominant cause of brain disease, and increasingly robs the person of memory, spatial orientation, language and reasoning, sense of time and place, and other devastating changes as it completely destroys the mind.

Dementia with Lewy Bodies (DLB)

Dementia with Lewy bodies shows under a microscope the senile plaques of Alzheimer's disease but with far fewer tangles. Lewy body dementia affects the areas of the brain that control thinking and movement functions. It is the second most prevalent form of progressive dementia after Alzheimer's disease. In some studies, it is believed to be the cause of dementia in up to 10% of patients in the elderly group. Patients with Lewy body dementia show a change in the brain cells that is normally associated with Parkinson's disease. The difference is that Lewy bodies, which are abnormal protein deposits, are typically concentrated in one part of the brain, whereas in Parkinson's, certain cells break down and die, and their effects can be widely distributed throughout the brain. The fluctuations in cognitive impairment, memory loss, and confusion, can be quite intense in Lewy body dementia; hallucinations and paranoia are frequent.

Vascular Dementia

Vascular dementia is seen in patients with recurring stroke and severe cell damage from disease of the small arteries to the central part of the brain. Vascular dementia is a common cause of dementia and is brought about by strokes. The symptoms of vascular dementia are similar to those of Alzheimer's disease. The most noticeable symptoms of this state include depression, epileptic seizures, acute confusion, hallucinations, delusions, physical and verbal aggression, and restlessness. A mixture of vascular dementia and Alzheimer's disease is more common, and a person with this combination can deteriorate further, even without suffering another stroke.

Parkinson's Disease Dementia

Parkinson's disease starts with problems in movement and is characterized by tremors, stiffness to the joints and limbs, and slowness of movement. There is also a problem with balance, and sufferers generally have difficulty walking. Dementia is common in the advanced stages of Parkinson's disease. It is different from Alzheimer's disease in that Parkinson's patients will suffer a slower rate of memory recall, whereas Alzheimer's patients won't remember anything. People with Parkinson's dementia tend to have more hallucinations. The loss of mobility and cognitive impairment contribute to the functional decline in Parkinson's patients.

Frontotemporal Dementia (FTD)

Frontotemporal dementia, or *Picks disease,* is a relatively uncommon type of dementia and is seen in 5–10% of all dementia patients. The key features are atrophy of the frontal and temporal lobes of the brain. The symptoms include prominent language changes such as the inability to name an object *(anomia)*, the inability to generate or comprehend language (aphasia), the tendency to repeat everything said to them (echolalia), and the tendency to repeat a word or phrase in an obsessive manner, without awareness *(perseverative speech)*. Many patients suffering from this type of dementia lose social skills and display inappropriate behaviour, lack of judgement, and an inability to understand.

Other Degenerative Disease Dementia

Chronic infections, such as *tuberculous meningitis* can also give rise to cognitive impairment. Other degenerative diseases, such as progressive *supranuclear palsy*, a Parkinson-like condition, are seen in patients with balance problems and trouble moving their eyes. Lou Gehrig's disease, or *amyotrophic lateral sclerosis* (ALS), is a degenerative disease that causes severe and progressive atrophy of muscles, and is associated with dementia. *Huntington's disease* is characterized by intense squirming movements, depression, and dementia. This disease attacks individuals in their early forties, fifties, or sixties.

Common Dementia Symptoms:

* Memory loss
* Challenges in performing regular and familiar tasks
* Feeling lost in familiar surroundings
* Losing sense of time and place
* Loss of language (common in the more advanced stages of dementia)
* Substantial decrease in judgement and comprehension
* Unable to solve problems or think intelligently
* Misplacing things
* Attitudes and behaviour changes
* Personality changes
* Loss of motivation

The 7 Stages of Alzheimer's disease

Alzheimer's disease begins long before severe cognitive decline and manifestations occur. It is suggested that the earlier the disease is detected, the longer the patient can maintain a quality of life. Dementia is characterized by the decline and breakdown of a person's mental functions and capabilities. Alzheimer's disease is still misdiagnosed in spite of its rampage and the fact that it is the primary cause of dementia.

A guideline is provided below to demonstrate seven different stages of Alzheimer's disease, to help individuals identify the symptoms and to embark on treatment and care sooner rather than later. Each stage displays different symptoms. Some patients do not go through all the stages. Rapid progression of the disease is more often caused by other diseases or other contributing factors. There is no one universal template for all Alzheimer's sufferers, since symptoms vary in every individual.

Stage 1:
At this stage, everything appears to be normal, and there are no notable signs of decline in mental, judgement, or reasoning capability. This stage can last for many years.

Stage 2:
There are mild cognitive problems, since Alzheimer's affects the part of the brain that stores memory. Memory lapse occurs, and thinking becomes compromised. It takes longer to remember words, places, or things, or to perform daily tasks the normal way. This stage might be associated with old age, and go unnoticed by family or friends.

Stage 3:
At this stage, there are noticeable cognitive issues, which are not part of aging. The part of the brain that is affected is the temporal lobe, which controls memory and language. The affected person will begin to sense that something is wrong, and others close to the individual will also begin to take notice of the marked changes.

Stage 4:
Moderate cognitive disability is demonstrated. A thorough medical exam can detect problems and other clear indications of impairment. At this stage, the frontal lobe, which is associated with short-term memory tasks such as planning or driving, is fully affected.

Stage 5:
More symptoms become very apparent. Family members seek help and care for their loved one and for themselves, as the disease has advanced to such a stage that the new behaviours are beyond their scope of management. This stage is characterized by memory loss, and confusion becomes more apparent. Delusions, hallucinations, depression, agitation, and sleepiness set in from major gaps in memory functions and cognitive ability. Families should start searching for long-term care facilities for their loved ones, to reduce the stress and worries on their daily lives.

Stage 6:
This is referred to as the late stage or severe Alzheimer's. The disease has been present for a number of years and, like cancer, has taken root and rendered its victim completely helpless.   This is the most emotionally turbulent stage for relatives, friends, and caregivers, seeing their loved ones in such distress. There is no magic pill to make them right. At this stage, the Alzheimer's sufferer is usually placed in long-term care to provide the extensive care necessary and to bring back some peace and normalcy to the lives of family members. In long-term care, the patient is under a 24/7 professional watch, with caregivers providing exceptional care. At this stage, the patient loses the ability to express their needs.

Their memories are severely impacted, and they can no longer recognize loved ones or remember anything of their lives. Language is unintelligible; they may become physically aggressive toward caregivers and are resistant toward basic care such as dressing, feeding, or bathing. Wandering is common and, if left unsupervised, the patient will wander off and get lost. People with Alzheimer's lose the ability to comprehend and can be agitated or paranoid. Other behaviours at this stage are difficulties in walking, difficulty swallowing and increasingly slower and more rigid movements.

Stage 7:
The individual is fully dependent on caregivers at this stage. The patient may even be bed-ridden and need caregivers to provide the activities of daily living, such as feeding, bathing, going to the bathroom, and medications. This is practically the final stage. The patient is not able to smile, movement is restricted, there are muscle contractures, and joint deformity occurs. Care around the clock is required. Pneumonia is the most frequent cause of death in Alzheimer's disease sufferers, followed by bedsores, stroke and heart disease, or cancer. The central nervous system functions are quite deteriorated, and organ failure is imminent in some cases.

Symptoms of Alzheimer's Disease

Dementia – This is a term used for a set of symptoms manifested by different brain disorders. People with dementia suffer impaired logical and cognitive functioning that interferes with their normal activities and relationships. The most common cause of dementia is Alzheimer's disease, commonly found in people over 60. The brain functions that are affected include memory, language, movement, behaviour, judgement, and abstract thinking.

Depression – Depression has a scientifically proven link to Alzheimer's disease. This is a mental disorder wherein a person exhibits a depressed mood, feelings of guilt, loss of interest in activities, disturbed sleep, loss of appetite, low energy, and poor concentration for a while. This can be brought about by traumatic events such as the death of a loved one, divorce, illness, or loss of a job. It can also be triggered by the use of certain medications and abuse of substances or alcohol. This disorder can be disabling, and may hinder a normal active life. Severe depression is a major cause of disability. Research has found a strong link between major depressive disorder and Alzheimer's related dementia.

Anxiety – Scientific research confirms that there is a connection between anxiety and Alzheimer's. Anxiety is a feeling of worry or apprehension that may be coupled with physical symptoms such as tense muscles, numbness, headache, trembling, excessive sweating, nausea, palpitations, and diarrhea. Anxiety disorders have been associated with irregular levels of neurotransmitters in the brain, the major organ affected by Alzheimer's disease. These neurotransmitters are essentially chemical messengers that move data from one nerve cell to the next.

Wandering – Researchers have classified wandering, in the case of Alzheimer's disease, as a very serious problem. It is often referred to as critical wandering, and is defined as decreased cognitive ability in an Alzheimer's patient who wanders away from supervised care.

Agitation – Agitation can be defined as a state of mind where there is increased tension and occurrences of emotional and physical irritability. This can be caused by drugs, alcohol, withdrawal, depression, hyperthyroidism, asthma, head injury, stress, lack of sleep, heart attack, or stroke. More often than not, the sufferers of Alzheimer's show agitation. The symptom usually shows up in the middle stages of the disease.

Aggression – Patients with Alzheimer's disease exhibit increased levels of aggression. This aggressive behaviour may be in the form of verbal acts such as shouting and name calling, or physical actions such as pushing or hitting. The behavioural symptom is due to the progressive decline of brain cells. Environmental factors can also provoke the symptom or make it worse. Patients can sometimes display out-of-character anger and frustration, which is disturbing to family and caregivers. Understanding the triggers can sometimes lessen the problems and increase safety.

Paranoia – Alzheimer's disease patients often suffer from paranoia. The primary symptom of paranoia is the gradual onset of delusions, which may end up lasting for a long time. The person afflicted by paranoia has feelings of suspiciousness, irritability, depression, distrust, and bitterness.

Hallucinations – Clinical data conclude that Alzheimer's disease patients suffer from hallucinations, which involve seeing things that are just not there. However, they are very realistic to the person who is awake and conscious. Hallucinations include a crawling sensation on the skin, hearing non-existent voices, and seeing lights or objects.

Keeping the Home Safe

"If I have to beat you up to keep you safe, that's just what I'll do.
It's this kind of regard for others that make me believe
I'd be a good politician."
Jarod Kintz

Safety in the home environment is very important in planning the care of individuals with Alzheimer's disease. A research team from Thomas Jefferson University reported that people with dementia, especially those in the third stage of the disease, are often compelled to act out in a definite and decisive manner. In their tangled minds, they are called to cook, chop things, or go on errands. Often, people who may be living alone, or with family or a caregiver, face serious and numerous safety risks. These risks include injuries from falls, coming in contact with sharp objects, consuming or inhaling dangerous substances, suffering burns from lighted stoves or getting scalded by boiling water, or just simply walking away from a protected environment and getting lost. Maintaining a safe environment is a major challenge for families and caregivers.

Maximizing home safety is simply done by using safe environmental strategies. It is predictable that the capabilities of the Alzheimer's patient will decline in the third stage of the disease. These individuals will continue to have difficulties moving through spaces, or they may want to move things around or even sample substances that look familiar. As a result of the erosion in faculties and abilities of the patient, families and caregivers need to periodically reassess the physical safety of the environment, and plan new approaches to maintain an accident-free space, in addition to providing intensive supervision and attention.

Keeping Loved Ones Safe

As in the words of Susan Elizabeth Phillips, *"I finally figured out that not every crisis can be managed. As much as we want to keep ourselves safe, we can't protect ourselves from everything. If we want to embrace life, we also have to embrace chaos."*

To keep your loved one with dementia safe is a cliché. Each person's bout with dementia is different. In the situation with my mother, we did all we could to keep her safe; but sadly, it turned out not to be the case. However, if it gives you any solace, I have discovered tips over the years from my experience as a caregiver, to help other caregivers and families to keep their loved ones safe. There are coping strategies in this chapter that may be helpful.

Behaviour

It is sometimes frustrating trying to get someone to understand you, let alone someone with dementia. Getting them to comply when they are acting up is difficult, and sometimes downright impossible. The first thing to keep in mind is the safety of the one in your care and, to some extent, to be mindful of your own safety. Sometimes you will have to give in to their stubbornness, and other times you will have to be firm. It is easier, however, for you to change your behaviour than to change the behaviour of your loved one.

Find ways to accommodate their wishes rather than getting embroiled in constant struggle. You can't win a fight, nor can you win the conversation, which has no direction or aim. Track down the cause of some changes in behaviour, as there may be a reason behind the patient's acting up. Keep a close vigil on the patient's well-being; you may discover that it's a change in medication that's causing dizziness or irritability, a change they may not be able to identify themselves.

Communication

A dementia patient who has behavioural issues makes verbal communication very challenging. He may not understand the spoken language, making it difficult to get the message across.

The following are tips to communicating more effectively:

1. Your loved ones are more likely to pick up on emotion, but only if these emotions are clearly expressed. Wear a big smile for them to see that you still love them. For example, if your mother is looking for her dead mother, trying to explain that she is not around anymore is pointless to a wounded mind. Instead, try to comfort her with an embrace.

2. Use touch to make sure that they are focused on you. Use simple phrases, and don't raise your voice because an answer was not forthcoming. Instead, repeat what you want to say, using very clear and specific terms.

3. Phrase questions that invite a yes or no answer. Be patient if you are not getting through. You may have to stop and try again at a later time.

4. A conversation with your loved one may not lead to the positive result that you hope for. Instead, do something to create a distraction, like offering something to eat or drink, or changing the topic altogether. The diversion is likely to be calming.

5. There may be certain times of the day when communication is more effective, such as after a nap or in the middle of the morning when the patient is likely to be mentally alert. Pay attention to the medications being used, to assess if they have positive or negative effects. Avoid communicating during a low point of interest or energy.

6. Keep other distractions to a minimum when talking to someone with dementia. Turn off the television and radio, and draw the blinds so that the patient is spared of distractions and can focus on what you are saying. They may not remember everything you say, but at least for the moment, they have only you to listen to.

7. If your loved one keeps asking you to repeat what you are saying, the problem may be impaired hearing. Poor hearing may cause agitation, and increase frustration. Bring this condition to your doctor's attention.

8. Have sufficient time to initiate a conversation. Your loved one needs time to gather his or her thoughts, and should not be interrupted when

speaking. Fill in the words if necessary; showing you are engaging in the conversation keeps them from getting frustrated and may mean a lot to them.

9. Delusional patients have difficulty separating facts from fiction. Don't simply dismiss what they are seeing as imaginary figments. Instead, offer comfort because, to them, what they are seeing is real. Dismissing their visions or attempting to persuade them that they are not real will only cause anxiety and agitation. Be aware of what they watch on the television or listen to on the radio. Unexpected news can trigger suppressed memories that surface as anxiety or frustration.

10. Physical problems, such as urinary tract infections, toothache, or pain, can trigger delusions. The patient may not be able to point to existing problems, and rather than making a coherent complaint about discomfort, he or she resorts to delusional behaviour. It is important to be attentive to everything they do; for example, stopping eating or staying away from foods they love may be brought about by a toothache.

Rage

A person may scream or use profanity, or be physical, from frustration or anxiety. A person who exhibits rage does so because there is no self-consciousness. Someone with dementia has no filter on behaviour and will express a full range of emotions.

But if you look at the situation in perspective, and see through the lens of delusional thinking that is affecting the patient, it may be easier for you to accept or put up with the emotional outbursts. Dealing with rage is not easy; it can drain you of energy and, if not handled correctly, may even compromise your own health. You love the patient enough to put up with episodes of rage, so seek proper help, and exercise tough love when necessary. Also look into medications, which may reduce this behaviour.

Sundowning

Sundowning is a common problem. It refers to the state of agitation that Alzheimer's sufferers slip into at night. If you have a sundowner on your hands, you may have to put up with sleepless nights. Be mindful that lack of proper sleep can affect your health and undermine the quality of care given to the patient.

Here are some tips to help you cope with your sundowner:

1. Keep the sundowner busy during the day so that he or she will fall asleep at night.

2. Instead of a day facility for your loved one, choose a place that offers care during the night. Remember, you are the caregiver, and your health is very important. A proper night's sleep or a healthy sleeping pattern is vital for you to properly and adequately deal with the patient.

3. Sometimes a combination of medicinal and behavioural therapy is necessary to calm your loved ones who may be out of control. I hope that you do not have to revert to strong sedation to calm the patient, because it takes away any mental alertness they may still have.

4. Take note of every new development or change. Observe the impact of drugs, and work closely with your doctor to get to the right combination of drugs that work best for the patient. This ensures that they stay more alert and are less prone to anxiety. Some caregivers balk at the thought of medicating their parent or spouse, but remember that you need sleep too. If the sundowner is under control, you will be able to get the necessary sleep.

Wanderers

Dementia sufferers often wander. Individuals may wander off when they get agitated or are frustrated with their condition or the way they interact with their environments. Sticking to a routine, or making sure that everything they need—such as glasses, TV remote, or Kleenex—is always in the same place, is helpful. Some wandering may be caused by delusions, which make it impossible for them to discern the difference between the pictures in their heads and the real world they live in.

The following may help to mollify or deter wandering:

1. Soften the lighting in the common areas where they are likely to hang out.

2. Lock all exit doors, making sure that these actions comply with the safety code for your environment, home, or building.

3. Disguise a door by hanging a poster over it so that it appears as an ordinary wall.

4. Place a black mat before the door; the mat may come across as a hole in the ground, and deter the patient from approaching that area.

5. Use plastic covers on door handles, such as those used to prevent children from opening doors. These plastic covers are slippery enough that a person needs to firmly grip the handle in order to open the door.

6. Simply placing a "Stop" sign on the door may be a sufficient deterrent.

7. Have the loved one wear an ID bracelet, sew name tags onto their clothes, or place a note with important details, such as name, address, and phone number, to help you track them when they are lost.

8. Place alarms on all doors to alert you when a door is opened. This may be necessary to rein in the determined wanderers when all other solutions have failed.

9. Have your loved one wear a tracking device such as a GPS. A tracking device is good for early-stage sufferers, who are unable to recall where they were heading to, or to be cognizant of where they are, when they stray away from their regular routes.

A wanderer is more likely to walk out in the direction of the door they have previously used. The patient may also attempt to go back to their former work-place, or decide they have to go grocery shopping to prepare meals for the family. Stay aware and listen for clues in their regular chatter.

Chapter -6-

Taking Control of Alzheimer's

"Nothing is impossible; the word itself says I'm possible."
Audrey Hepburn

An Early Handle on Alzheimer's Disease

Alzheimer's disease is a progressive, invasive, degenerative, and irreversible neurological disorder. It inflicts physical suffering on its prey, and robs the individual of willpower and motivation. The disease is characterized by gradual and constant changes that worsen as time passes. Heavy emotions, such as self-pity, despair, and guilt, follow on the heels of finding out the diagnosis. There are a number of drugs that provide a decent level of relief from symptoms. However, disease imposes a heavy burden on those who undertake the care of the afflicted and are committed to keeping them sound and safe.

There is research that seeks to find more effective drugs to treat the disease. Tremendous strides have been made. Patients are enjoying a better quality of life and are living longer. The trick is to catch the symptoms or changes, no matter how small they are, in time, before they get progressively more serious. Memory lapses may be symptomatic of old age, but not in all cases. Get your loved one tested early during a routine visit to your doctor. While there is no cure for the disease, there is hope that the decline can be slowed down.

The Sooner the Better for Caregivers

Learn as much as you can about the disease. There are Alzheimer's associations and organizations in your community that will provide the necessary information to better prepare you. Understanding the process of the disease will help in planning the transition, for both families and caregivers. A caregiver should avoid thinking that he or she is alone on this journey. No matter how dedicated a family member, friend, or caregiver you are, you will need help, even at the first stages of the disease. Support is very important in caring for an Alzheimer's disease victim because, when you get down to it, we are all victims of a cruel disease. Escape the reality at hand. Get help for daily activities such as driving, preparation of meals, or even running errands like banking and shopping. Find support to provide a consistent structure for daily activities.

Taking First Steps

Spotting the disease early improves the chances of benefitting from treatment. I outlined the various stages of Alzheimer's to help you identify disturbing symptoms when they occur. Don't rule out unusual behaviour. Take immediate action and get the loved one tested by your physician. Early detection and diagnosis improves the odds of profiting from treatment, and reduces the emotional and physical toll arising from dealing with the unknown and the inexplicable, on the patient and the family.

Early action better preserves the patient's brain function, and may even give them years of productivity and independence. It also gives the person the opportunity to be involved in planning and making decisions for the future, including personal care and financial and legal matters. Individuals who are diagnosed early may be fortunate enough to participate in clinical tests, where scientists test and determine the safety, effectiveness, and side effects of new drugs and treatments. All in all, with more time on their hands, the afflicted individual and family can find high-quality support and care services, lessening the burden on them.

Is It Really Old Age?

No one likes to find out that there is something wrong with them. It is necessary for the person manifesting symptoms of the disease to be evaluated by a doctor or physician; studies show that doctors are able to diagnose Alzheimer's disease with about 90% accuracy. They do so through a simple process of elimination to rule out other health problems, which may have the same symptoms. Once Alzheimer's is suspected, the family doctor should refer the patient to specialists. Specialists will use bio markers to confirm the diagnosis and come up with possible treatments. *(A biomarker is a substance in the body that can be measured to reliably indicate the presence or absence of a disease, or even just the risk for developing a disease.)*

For example, amyloid beta (AB or beta-amyloid protein accumulation) is a major biomarker for the onset of Alzheimer's. A high glucose level is a biomarker for diabetes; elevated cholesterol is a biomarker for heart disease. Alzheimer's disease begins long before severe cognitive decline manifests. New procedures are in place to detect and diagnose the disease early, long before dementia develops. Unfortunately, in spite of strides in research and technological advances in diagnostic techniques, there is still a high incidence of misdiagnosis in the early stages.

Using Diet to Maintain Brain Health

Alzheimer's sneaks up on the unsuspecting as a thief in the dark, and snatches the minds of its victims, slowly and gradually robbing them of their faculties and identity through profound changes in the brain. We have within our power the capability to fight this disease. A healthy lifestyle plays an important role in the prevention and treatment of this condition.

There is a feeling of empowerment from safeguarding the health of your brain and the brains of your loved ones. Harvest the power of choice to make life-altering changes to stop this disease in its tracks. By adopting preventative strategies like dietary changes and healthy foods, you can rebuff Alzheimer's or even delay the onset of symptoms for many years. Nutritional science research has identified trends in food consumption that appear to lead to lower incidence of Alzheimer's' disease and cognitive decline. A proper diet assists in maintaining normal bodily functions, while poor diets have been linked to certain diseases.

Diets containing a significant quantity of vitamins have been associated with a healthy brain, while diets that are high in cholesterol increase the risk of stroke and brain damage. An effective combination is a healthy diet and exercise. The best diets for a healthy brain are those that contain omega-3 fatty acids, fruits, vegetables, and whole grains. There are detailed studies on the sources of good and bad diets, which you can easily access online.

According to statistics, we can lower the occurrence of Alzheimer's disease by 5%, by the year 2030. This is significant when the cost to treat Alzheimer's disease patients is phenomenal.

Select your foods wisely. Reading the label is a guide to better understanding how the choices you make can impact changes in the brain. Any changes you make toward good food consumption practices greatly benefit you and your loved ones, now and in the future. Adopt a brain-healthy diet. This is described in a later chapter.

The Fortitude of Caregivers

"Courage is the most important of all the virtues because without courage, you can't practice any other virtue consistently."
Maya Angelou

Courage

Alzheimer's disease is relentless. Family members, friends, companions, and caregivers get emotionally and financially exhausted. Yet they have to step up to the plate; they have to dig deep within themselves to ensure that their helpless loved ones get continuing quality care. This is by no means a small task that is imposed on the family members. They have to care for and advocate on behalf of the victim, rally to hospitals, anticipate phone calls from care facilities, call for emergency assistance, and be at their bedside, and yet still find time and energy to balance their own lives. These are remarkable acts of courage. It is also equally important that caregivers develop an awareness and understanding of the disease so that they have tolerance for the patient's feeling. A caregiver with courage and confidence means a happier and healthier patient.

Don't Take It Personally

In the advanced stages of the disease, the afflicted are often weak and vulnerable. Tolerance and persistence are necessary and important to attending to their physical needs. There are times when your loved one, either at home or in a nursing facility, will resort to irritating conduct that upsets family or caregivers. Know that it is no fault of theirs; they are unaware of what they are doing.

You may be prone to be critical or judgemental of such behaviour; but quite frankly, this attitude will not resolve the problem or dim the intolerable anguish you may feel at seeing your loved one in such unmanageable distress. Even the best caregivers will feel frustrated and underrated under such circumstances. They may feel that their efforts are all in vain. Think of this: Even if the patient wants to thank you for your help, they are completely devoid of the ability to articulate the words or to make a gesture of appreciation.

If it makes you feel better, recall those times when the loved one was at his or her best, and think of the impact they have had. Dip into the past to remember what your mother, father, brother, sister, aunt, or uncle once stood for. At the same time, you need to develop the strength, courage, and fortitude to step away from the emotional connection. Sticking to a regular routine makes it easier. Remember that you can ask for help from your medical teams, fellow caregivers, or community support circles. You do not have to carry this burden alone.

Chapter -7-

Unchartered Territory:
Balancing the Rigors of Care with Asking for Help

*"In the heart of every caregiver is a knowing that we are all connected.
As I do for you, I do for me."*
Tia Walker

The love and attention, given by caregivers to their loved ones suffering from dementia and Alzheimer's, plays a pivotal role in helping to slow the decline of the patient.

Studies by John Hopkins University in Baltimore, and Utah State University, suggest that a close and intimate relationship between patient and caregiver gives those with Alzheimer's a noticeable advantage over those who are not as lucky. The emotional connection is as important as the drugs prescribed to slow the disease. These more fortunate patients manage to retain their mind and brain functions for longer than those who don't have family caregivers.

This very same study looked into the relationship between 167 pairs of patients and caregivers. Those who were being looked after by their spouses declined most slowly; and the scores, which measure changes over time, were similar to those of patients in clinical trials for FDA-approved Alzheimer's drugs known as acetylcholinesterase inhibitors.

Yet the toll on the caregivers can be as punitive as the disease itself, and in view of this discovery of how loving caregiving can make such a substantial difference, it is crucial for you, as the caregiver, to know when to give yourself a break and when to ask for help.

At the beginning, you may feel energized and strong enough to go it alone. Caregiving in the initial stages of Alzheimer's is effortless compared to the demands of the end stages. The early stages are the easiest to deal with. Remember that you aren't the only one in the world who is experiencing these uncharted waters. Taking care of someone is hard work. Taking care of someone with Alzheimer's is even more difficult. I know from experience.

Don't allow yourself to get overwhelmed. Always refer back to the wisdom in this book, as it will be your guide and companion. Making the required changes to your life and routine immediately, before your loved one experiences complete memory loss, ensures that the journey will be much more straightforward and considerably easier to handle. Sticking your head in the sand will make it extremely tough for everyone. This map to compassionate caregiving of patients with Alzheimer's, and those who may be afflicted with dementia, is designed to be your guide along the painful journey. It is written specifically to help you, the caregiver, to prepare, organize, de-stress, and equip yourself with the tools, strategies, and skills you will need in order to minimize the physical, mental, and emotional upheavals that all involved will experience.

Three Stages of Caregiving

"I realized how truly hard it was, really, to see someone you love change right before your eyes. Not only is it scary, it throws your balance off as well."
Sarah Dessen

Early-Stage Caregiving

You need to know that there are three different stages of caregiving. The first stage, early-stage caregiving, is the easiest. There is no guarantee as to how long this stage will last. Don't think negatively, because there is a chance that this stage will last until your loved one passes. Even if it is a very small chance, it is still there, so keep your hopes up for your own sake. Hope is an antidote to despair and fear, which we will talk about more in the next chapter.

Yet this doesn't mean that you don't need to face the illness head-on and be honest with yourself about what to expect. Denial can be dangerous, especially when your loved one is first diagnosed. He or she may not even know that they have symptoms of Alzheimer's. It's up to you to gently break the truth to them.

The sooner they begin receiving treatment, the better. Denial can happen because a person is not ready to be responsible for the one suffering with Alzheimer's. Whether you are ready or not, you are smack dab in the middle of something called LIFE, which at this point in time has served you a low-ball. If you are willing to make the best of it, remain positive, and accept that your loved one has Alzheimer's, you can grow and learn a lot from this experience. This can be embarrassing and frustrating because of social stigmas surrounding the disease. Your goal, as caregiver, is to keep your own emotions in check so that you can be strong enough to help and encourage them through this rough time.

The afflicted will need emotional support as well as help planning for the future. You will need to help your loved one with their memory by reminding them about appointments, medication times and, most of all, recollection of people, places, and things. Encouragement is essential, and giving your loved one options of activities or support groups to get involved with is helpful and necessary. At this stage, you may not need much help. But there are no two ways about it; it does get tougher.

Middle-Stage Caregiving

The second stage, or middle-stage caregiving, requires a much greater responsibility. You will need to learn to be more patient and compassionate. You are more greatly involved and need to interact more frequently with other members of the caregiving team. These other members may be the husband or wife, a parent, a close relative, or a sibling. All caregivers and those responsible for the patient's welfare should agree on decisions about patient care. Be aware of sibling rivalry, burnt-out spouses, or the burden of having to travel long distances regularly to your loved ones. Such circumstances can adversely affect both the patient and the caregiver. You won't necessarily feel like it all the time, but remember that love is a choice. The more you love, the easier it becomes. Just remember that love is power, and it brings healing, not only to the one you love but to yourself as well.

At this point, don't be afraid to ask friends and family for help. There are also plenty of community-wide resources available, so seek those out as well. Changes in behavior will be more apparent. Brush up on the necessary change management strategies. When the patient is asking a question, and sometimes repeatedly, don't just listen to the words. Pay as much, if not more, attention to the emotion behind the question. Your loved one may just need additional reassurance and care.

Daily care needs will multiply; at this point, you will need to be more patient and gentle. Don't talk as fast as you would normally, and show compassion through your eyes and voice. Don't be afraid to look your loved one directly in the eyes. The eyes are the windows to the soul, and they will feel your compassion resonating in their soul even if they do not understand what you are saying.

Late-Stage Caregiving

Late-stage caregiving can be painfully traumatic. Be prepared for it. Expect to be needed at all times by your loved one. They will need help with eating, walking, personal care, medical care, and communicating. At this point, they are just like infants who need constant care, compassion, and patience.

Like babies who don't understand your words, they will understand other forms of caregiving such as spending time with them, reading together, listening to music together, and going for walks if they are physically able to do so. Babies require constant care, and so do those with end-stage Alzheimer's. If you are not able to provide quality full-time care at home, it may be necessary to move your loved one into a personal care home at this final stage. It won't be an easy decision, and that is why I'm attempting to prepare you for this ahead of time.

You may say right now that you will never let this happen. But once you become overwhelmed, you will start thinking about it at that point. Trust me, it happens to the best of us. Instead of waiting until the last minute, begin researching now about different personal care homes. There are many differences, and you may find one to be much better than another.

Plan in advance when and how to move a loved one with dementia to a care facility. Conduct research on care facilities well ahead of time to ensure that you arrive at a sensible and well-thought-out decision that would be best for the patient. When you've your back against the wall, it isn't easy to make a sensible and rational plan. Look for a facility that offers individual care, to ensure that the patient is consistently attended to and supervised.

Stress Check

"Whatever you want to do, do it now; there are only so many tomorrows."
Michael Landon

If you are overburdened by caregiving, and feel stressed out, don't add to the emotional weight on you by feeling guilty. Guilt is unproductive and erodes your optimism and energy. You are doing the best you can at this moment in time. If you need to, take a break. Ask another family member to take over for a day or two.

Besides having other family member's help, you may need to create a routine schedule of caregiving. To arrange a realistic caregiving formula is to divide care into bite-size pieces, so that you don't cave into overwhelm. There are many, many details that need to be handled, and the tasks will change with the progressive onset of the disease. There's no doubt in the world that this will be difficult for you and your family members. The last thing you want is to overthink everything, because this will put a heavy weight upon your soul.

The best way to lighten the load of personal care for your loved one throughout the day is to create a routine. Beginning any routine is challenging, no matter what it's about or who it's for. Even a routine for your own life will be difficult at the beginning. In time, you become used to it.

Once both you and your loved one get used to a routine, which you will be able to plan and write out ahead of time, you will be able to add more activities into the schedule. You may even decide to divide this schedule into smaller and briefer sections. Timing may not be of importance as long as everything gets done. Firstly, arrange sections into daily care, personal care, and medical care.

For example, daily care will include making meals, spending time together, and activities. Personal care would include bathing, dressing, and grooming. As part of the tasks involved in medical care, you will need to give them their medications, take them to appointments, and ensure that they feel okay, both emotionally and physically. Use different color markers to denote the different types and timing of activities, and check each item off as it is completed. Carefully organizing and structuring your daily caregiving activities helps decrease your stress levels, helps you maintain control, and calms your spirits.

How to Find Help

"One of the greatest barriers to connection is the cultural importance we place on 'going it alone.' Somehow we've come to equate success with not needing anyone. Many of us are willing to extend a helping hand, but we're very reluctant to reach out for help when we need it ourselves. It's as if we've divided the world into 'those who offer help' and 'those who need help.' The truth is that we are both."
Brené Brown

If you are a caregiver to someone with Alzheimer's, you are not alone. It's vital to remember this, especially during those times when you feel like throwing in the towel. Your loved one needs you more than ever right now. Put yourself in their shoes. Wouldn't you want someone who loves you to take care of you without feeling exhausted or angry? Having a support network that you can count on is a necessary help during this time. Your own well-being is just as important as your loved ones.

There are various workshops, training classes, and certification courses that you can easily find online. There are also books, audio books, CDs, and DVDs that you can purchase to help you along. There are many online and community-wide support groups available as well. Begin searching through internet sources. Also, ask your loved one's health care provider for additional advice on where to get assistance and support.

Online sources such as www.webmd.com have more than general knowledge for you to research and look through. Web MD online offers information about where to find the help you need. Professional associations also have plenty of information, support, and educational resources available. The Alzheimer Society of Canada is dedicated to providing help to people with Alzheimer's disease and other forms of dementia, and to their caregivers. Education, resources, and support are available in every province across Canada and in over 150 local communities. The better prepared you are, the more confident you will feel in your own ability to give compassionate care to your loved one who desperately needs your help.

Bridging the Emotional Divide

Family members, including yourself, should stay in contact with the loved one, even if they cannot connect through conversation. Emotional bonds are the strongest connectors, especially within families. If everyone in the family will stay together and stick this out for the long run, it will ultimately help everyone to stay stronger and emotionally healthy. This emotional health is necessary for a sense of well-being, which will give each person the extra strength needed to care for the patient.

It will also be helpful if the family spends some time together by eating meals, going to church, or attending other events. Be intentional in your desire to connect and stay connected with each other. It won't just happen. Don't expect the next person to plan an outing, pay for dinner, or drive everyone around on his or her own.

Be the initiator, ask for help, and divvy out to each person his or her specific assignment. Make it clear what it is that you want to do in terms of a family outing. If you want to have dinner at home, have one or two people cook the meal while everyone else spends time together talking, listening to music, or watching television. When everyone becomes involved with the process, it will be more difficult for them to say no to the caregiver, who may request help from them in the future.

Chapter -8-

Coping With Emotional Turmoil

"Hiding my pain and acting strong, afraid to cry and show my tears,
I struggle with all this years later."
Erin Merryn

Caregivers will be dealing with a lot of emotions. This chapter offers techniques and suggestions on how to cope with the stress of caring for your loved one with Alzheimer's.

Expressing Emotions

Emotional turmoil will increase with time. How rough the going gets depends on how you handle your own emotions, how well you take care of yourself, and how you cope if you feel overwhelmed. Taking care of a patient creates a different bundle of stresses from the ones you experience in daily life. It is not as if, by being caregiver to a person with dementia, life will spare you from its highs and lows. On the contrary, at times you will feel so burdened that you'll want to collapse to your knees.

As a caregiver, accept that you will run through the gamut of emotions, and the strength of those feelings will be intensified. Firstly, you may experience denial. Recognize, however, that denial is not an emotion; it's a choice. In choosing denial, your heart and mind will feel overwhelmed with negative feelings such as anger, depression, and anxiety. Alternatively, if you have the courage to accept the truth of what is really happening, it will be easier to handle these same emotions when they show up.

Acceptance or denial does not really spare your heart from feeling as if it has been cut into a thousand pieces. As soon as you hear the diagnosis of Alzheimer's, you are likely to feel a punch in the gut and several unforgiving cuts to the heart. Anger and fear can rise up quickly, right before you attempt to deny that it's happening. Denial and fear work together, and they work against you, not for you. If you continue to be in denial, every time you see your loved one, anger may rear its ugly head. At this point, you are afflicted by a bundle of emotions—anger, fear, denial, depression—running headlong into each other.

Understanding that you may unravel when you begin to accept the harsh reality of the situation, is a truth in itself. You have to be real with yourself, especially when taking care of someone you love, who will increasingly depend on you. Don't beat yourself up for not being able to accept the diagnosis immediately. Such a reality cleaves your world and that of the patient's, and nothing will ever be the same again.

Forgive yourself if you need more time to come to grips with the situation. At the same time, understand that there is someone who needs you, your help, and your unconditional love. After you work through this process of healing, and the sobering honest truth, you will gradually be released from the pain, and you will get to a point where you will feel freer than you've ever felt in your life. This freedom occurs partly because you have come through the burning trials of a firestorm, and also because you now have the tools to deal with future heartache and agony. This is the stage where you are regaining control. You will grow much stronger, both mentally and emotionally, by working through the problem rather than going around it. As in all case, remember that the truth will set you free. Acceptance won't automatically heal your heart. But it is the first step to bringing the broken pieces back together. When you accept the truth, harsh and unrelenting though it may be, your heart feels free, as if heavy chains have dropped, because you are no longer lying to yourself. Deception creates some of the worst pains in this world because all that is really happening is that you are postponing the inevitable moment of pain. The way to accept your emotions is to open your heart, and feel the pain and through the pain. Be courageous, and allow yourself to fully embrace the emotions and the pain that are assailing you.

Maybe you don't need a deep healing because you have been expecting this diagnosis, and maybe you began grieving before this point. Either way, it's vital that you learn how to express your emotions and let them rise to the surface. Holding them in or burying them in your unconscious, no matter how convenient that might be, is detrimental to your health and manifests in insidious stress. It's vital for you to remain as stress-free as possible for your own well-being.

At this point, let's review some popular ways of expressing the human heart, which you can implement once you accept the truth of your new reality.

Methods of Coping

"The truth will set you free, but first it will make you miserable."
James A. Garfield

Before you can implement coping methods, you have to first acknowledge that you are under extreme stress. Many caregivers adopt a stoic role and keep a stiff upper lip. But the cracks in the face soon manifest in the form of getting irritable easily, being easily forgetful, not being able to sleep, withdrawal from contact with others, and becoming reclusive and losing interest in hobbies or pastimes. Be mindful and conscious that you don't become overburdened, overwhelmed, or exhausted to the point of burnout. When you fall ill, who is going to look after the patient? It's a sobering thought, isn't it?

Crying – Don't try to act strong when you know deep inside you aren't. Just let go. Even the strongest of us cry from time to time. Let your tears out. At this point, you may feel that you'll never feel whole ever again, but if you bottle up your emotions, you will eventually do much more than cry. At some point, you could have a breakdown. Instead of tears, you may yell in anger, or the buried stress could lead to a heart attack. You may even resort to violence and physically hurt someone because the repressed feelings need to find an outlet, somehow and somewhere.

If you feel like you cannot cry, scream out loud instead, but make sure that no one is around. Do it while driving if you can; go to a wide open space where no one can hear you. Screaming releases pent up emotions. You may find it hard to let go—what may first come out may be just a squeak—but give yourself permission to feel the pain, the anger, and the frustration. There are people in the world who have vowed to never shed a tear ever again, and since the mind is so powerful, their vow is so deeply buried in their subconscious that they can't ever force themselves to cry out their pain. If you fall into this category, screaming in private is a great source of relief. If this doesn't work, try punching a pillow.

Journaling – Writing in a journal or typing on your computer are healthy, creative, and beneficial ways to release your emotions. Write about your experiences, feelings, and the things that others have said and done that frustrate you. Review your writings to see the common thread that runs within, and see how you can find solutions to those gripes. Learn from your experiences so that you can be ultimately stronger.

Journaling is especially helpful should you need to express your point of view to a person who has hurt you, but who you are unwilling to confront directly. Your journal entries are, however, private; they are not meant to be shown to anyone. Just write as if you were going to give it to the offending party. Then delete it, set it afire, or tear it into pieces and flush it down the toilet, but don't send it. Alternatively, use the "Empty Chair Technique." Place a chair in front of you. Imagine that the hurtful person is sitting on the chair, and take that occasion to vent as loudly and as vehemently as you want, as if the person were really in your presence. You are the only person you can change, and this technique is shaped to let off steam in a safe and non-confrontational way, without hurting anyone.

Expressing Creativity – Creative expression is a powerfully wonderful way to heal the heart. When you are using your creative faculties, your focus is no longer on yourself or your pain. You are focusing outward, which eliminates much of that morbid introspective state we tend to fall into when we are in emotional pain. It does not matter what you do, whether it be to write a poem, story, or autobiography, or to make a scrapbook, paint a picture, design on your computer, bake cupcakes, play a musical instrument, dance, or chill by listening to music. Through any of these forms, you will have expressed yourself in a positive and constructive way, and had fun at the same time.

Grounding Through Meditation/Prayer – Meditation and prayer are not the same, but they are related. Although they are spiritual practices, it doesn't mean that you have to be an overtly spiritual person to take advantage of these coping methods. Meditation may seem strange to some, but it doesn't have to be. It's a form of deep breathing combined with a relaxed mind. You just need to find a quiet, comfortable place where you can be alone for at least 15 minutes. First, you must clear your mind of all anxious thoughts. Begin breathing in through your nose, and exhale through your mouth. If troublesome thoughts surface, don't force them away. Let them flow away, like a passing cloud in the sky.

When your mind is in a quiet, meditative place, you will be able to hear your inner voice much more clearly. Meditation is really about quieting the overactive intellectual mind, so that you can hear the voice of your soul and your intuition.

Prayer is not just about speaking words in church, a temple, or a mosque. Prayer is a two-way street. It's asking for help, and it also requires that you be able hear the answers or what is being said back to you. Those answers are only heard through the soft voice of your intuition, and you have to create those circumstances under which you can hear those soft whispers clearly. This is not something you can do if your mind is always in the way. Meditation is a bridge to prayer as much as prayer is a bridge to meditation, and as such, they both work hand in hand. If you have trouble clearing your mind before meditating, a short prayer will help you get into the right state so you can meditate in peace. If you are losing faith in the power of prayer, meditation will help re-establish the connection with all life and the sense of a bigger power than you.

Counseling and Support Groups – Counseling and support groups offer safe spaces for you to get your emotions out into the open, while also obtaining the support and guidance you require to deal with them. Deadly emotions such as guilt and rage, and suicidal ideas, fatigue, having difficulties making decisions, and physical symptoms, such as headaches, pain, and stomach problems, are major signs that you need counseling. Many people use counseling as a deterrent or preventative measure. Others wait until they are in total disarray or are at the point of imploding. Please don't wait until you feel as if you cannot even wake up in the mornings. Try everything you can before you allow extreme hopelessness to settle in your heart.

Feeling helpless is normal, but believe wholeheartedly that you are not alone. It will definitely feel as if the moorings have been cut and you are afloat in a stormy sea, on first discovering the cruel diagnosis. Not only does the patient need you at that point in time, you too need to reach out for help. You have a two-fold challenge before you. You need to understand the changes that the patient is undergoing, and his or her own turbulent emotions, and you need to come to grips with your own turmoil. A counselor can help you learn to identify the transformations that are taking place; such knowledge will reduce your stress dramatically.

A counselor may also recommend group therapy, as well as support groups or training in behaviour management strategies and problem-solving skills, out-side of the counseling atmosphere. Group therapy is a great way to meet people, connect with others, and gain all of the advice that you can, based on real experiences of real people who have been there and are going through it right now. Support groups will do the same things for you, and you may find that support groups are more convenient, depending upon your situation, your location, and the timing of the meetings.

Don't skip out on all these resources. Studies show that a spousal caregiver, who seeks individual and family therapy, support groups, and counseling, is less prone to depression and illnesses, and is able to postpone placing the patient in a nursing home, for upward of 18 months. These are 18 precious, extra months that you earn by taking care of yourself first.

Chapter -9-

The Stress of the Afflicted

"In the flush of love's light, we dare be brave.
And suddenly we see that love costs all we are
and will ever be. Yet it is only love which sets us free."
Maya Angelou

The patient in your care should be involved, mobile, and active. This chapter recognizes that mobility and exercises vary according to the stage that the patient is in. But in the early stages, the patient should stay involved with friends and family as much as possible.

Coping with Depression of the Afflicted

It's easy for the afflicted to become depressed. Their brains are failing to function properly, but they may not recognize that they are down in the dumps. For those who are still cognizant, they become susceptible to depression when they become aware of their progressive decline. Figures from the US-based Center for Disease Control show that 50% of older patients with Alzheimer's fall prey to depression; roughly 25% of them sink into a major depression.

If your loved one seems depressed in spirit, do everything you can to bring joy back into their life. Many times, they need companionship. They might be lonely living on their own. Even if it's a married couple, where one has been diagnosed with Alzheimer's, it can be very difficult for them to communicate and understand one another without help.

Alzheimer's is not a plague that requires that the patients be quarantined and kept out of the world. The patients still desire to be around family and friends, just as much as the healthy do. It's crucial that you help the Alzheimer's patient stay in contact with close friends and family members. Keeping active is a panacea to stave off depression and hopelessness. As long as your loved one is able to live life, help them get out there to live it—fully, thoroughly, and gratefully. Their brains might have lost power, but their spirits have not. When there is life, there is hope. Put yourself in their shoes, and do for them what you would want someone to do for you if you were diagnosed with the same medical problem.

Staying Active

For an Alzheimer's patient, staying active and retaining mobility is important for a number of reasons. For one, physical activity wards off negative emotions. It helps them to connect with others who enjoy the same activities, hobbies, and exercises. Secondly, physical exercise is very beneficial in the early stages of the disease because it increases blood flow to the brain, which ultimately increases healthy brain cells.

It's not guaranteed, but exercise may give the afflicted the ability to remain in the early stage of Alzheimer's for a much longer time than is the average observed in the majority of patients. Thirty minutes of regular exercise daily gets the body releasing the feel-good endorphins, which helps with pain and anxiety. Physical exercise doesn't have to be challenging in order to work well for the elderly. Aerobic activity increases both oxygen and blood flow to the brain, and can help reduce brain cell loss while maintaining muscle strength and joint flexibility, so that the patient may be able to cope independently for as long as possible.

The elderly may enjoy activities such as gardening, swimming, walking, bowling, and even seated exercises that can be done from home; but those in the earlier stages of Alzheimer's should be encouraged to be as mobile as possible. They are likely to significantly benefit from gentle forms of Chinese martial arts such as tai chi and qi gong, which combine gentle and simple physical movements and postures with deep breathing. These disciplines were first created as self-defense forms, but the gentle movements have been shown to positively impact mind, body, and spirit, and they strengthen balance, stability, and agility.

Tai chi involves many moving postures and is a form of moving meditation that focuses the person fully in the moment, and by so doing relieves emotional and mental stress. Qi gong can be practiced standing or sitting, and the key is to combine the physical movements with breathing, because it is through the breath that the body heals and re-energizes. Seated exercises are best for the later stages of the disease, when the patient won't be able to move around as much and is at greater risk of falling.

Maintaining a Healthy Weight

Maintaining a healthy weight involves more than just exercise. Many patients don't eat enough to remain healthy over the long term. They can lose too much weight even if they have a good nutritious diet. Their sense of smell and taste lessen with time, and the sensory deprivation makes food unappetizing or unpalatable to them. Further, they suffer indigestion or have problems with chewing, all of which can be exacerbated by the side effects of certain medications.

Their potential inability to handle utensils properly can be problematic. Delay the inevitable with strength training exercises; even simple exercises that just strengthen the fingers, hands, and arms are vital. Alzheimer's patients may even forget to eat, but don't mistake it as a willful refusal on their part and take out your anger on them. As the caregiver, it is important to be fully cognizant of the changes that will take place, so that you can remain centred and grounded at all times. This is the reason I am writing this book as a simple, one-stop guide for all caregivers. I hope you will keep this with you at all times for a quick and easy reference.

To be brutally honest, it does get worse over time. In the late stages of the disease, it's possible that the patient will spit food out, get up and walk around during mealtimes, and flat out refuse to eat. There isn't too much that you can do except encourage them, eat with them, add extra flavours and sweeteners to meals, and encourage them to exercise to burn enough calories. Burning calories through exercise is a good way to stimulate their hunger so that they will want to eat.

If the loved one is too thin, he or she may need to drink nutritional drinks and eat snacks throughout the day. If they lose weight while suffering from diabetes, there are special nutritional drinks and snacks, such as Glucerna, a low-sugar nutritional drink designed for people with diabetes. Maintaining a healthy weight can help prevent other common illnesses among the elderly, such as stroke, high blood pressure, heart attack, diabetes, cancer, arthritis, glaucoma, sleep changes, and osteoporosis.

Therapeutic Pursuits

Besides maintaining a healthy weight, there are other therapeutic activities and hobbies that promote well-being, decrease depression and stress, amongst many other advantages. Hopefully, it has become apparent that you will have a much easier time in caring for someone with Alzheimer's if you promote overall health in every area: physical, emotional, and mental. In the first stages of the disease, dance, art, and music are enjoyable activities that can help them to fight off depression and anxiety. You may decide to take your loved one to a concert or symphony, or carve out time to listen to music together at home.

Music promotes emotional healing and increases relaxation. Arts and crafts are also very popular amongst the elderly community. They feel a sense of connection when they pursue these activities together with friends. Light and easy dances can ease stress and burn calories at the same time.

Dancing may not be easy for those in the later stages of Alzheimer's. However, if you have a difficult time getting the patient out of the house, try to begin certain activities in the home first. Use a YouTube video that teaches easy dances; begin doing them yourself first, and invite the patient to join in. Try doing some simple arts and crafts as well. You may even enjoy yourself more than you expected.

Singing familiar songs together is also a great way to show you care, and it helps you to forget about the miseries of life. Find out what types of songs your loved one likes by playing a few songs from the era of time that they were brought up in. Writing and journaling are also great ways for the afflicted to deal with stressful situations and emotions. While they still can, encourage them to write in a diary, write poems, or write letters to friends and family to create keepsakes that will remind the survivors of them.

Creating Treasured Memories

Creating deep emotional ties is important for the family and friends of those with dementia. When it happens, you are painfully aware that your loved one's time on earth is finite and is shortened with the passing of each day. Many family members and friends wait until it's too late to connect and bond with those who are afflicted the disease. Once the loved one is in the final stage of dementia, it is too late, and the ones who survive are left with inconsolable regret and pain. Time is not a friend to those of you with loved ones suffering from this cruel disease. Make the most of the moments that you have, and do not postpone till tomorrow what you can do today to share a smile or laughter with your loved ones.

Do your best to create memories of joy and love instead of pain and frustration. Watch a funny movie together, take plenty of pictures, have fun eating out, and plan outings regularly. Plan a road trip and enjoy visiting destinations that you had hoped to get to "one day." The reality is that "one day" has arrived, and you must leverage these fleeting moments because, once they are gone, they stay gone and lost.

Don't allow your own frustration and negative emotions to show in front of the patient when he or she doesn't respond with the same enthusiasm as you hope and expect. You may have put a lot of care into designing a fun and interesting outing, but if your loved one is feeling tired, you may have to cut the trip short. You may feel unappreciated, but recognize that if they could, they would want to stay out as much as possible, but their minds and bodies are increasingly outside their control.

You, on the other hand, as the caregiver, have intact faculties. Exercise self-control to keep your sharp remarks in check, and deliberately and consciously choose love and compassion instead of anger. The patient needs to feel love from you, and his or her spirit can feel anger or negativity emanating from within your soul, even if the loved one can no longer articulate or understand you fully.

There are various alternative therapies to create memories. Family members can connect through art therapy, where the stricken paint and create works that express their creativity and help them focus, increasing self-confidence. Music therapy, light therapy, or sensory stimulation through taking a walk in the woods, are advocated as enhancing the enjoyment of the patient.

Chapter -10-

The Burden on Caregivers

"I promise you nothing is chaotic as it seems.
Nothing is worth diminishing your health.
Nothing is worth poisoning yourself into stress, anxiety, and fear."
Steve Maraboli

There's a chance that you may be too tired and stressed out to even realize how burned out you really are. You continue to run on fumes, or what is also known as adrenaline. Adrenaline is pumped out by a body that is required to undergo an enormous amount of pressure and strain. The bio-chemical is an endorphin, or the body's natural pain reliever. It is released by the adrenal glands and, once it is forcibly released, it will continue to be released unless the person decides to give the body a rest.

Caregiver Burnout

"It is not how much you do, but how much love you put in the doing."
Mother Theresa

Have you had trouble getting a full night's sleep? Are you getting enough restorative sleep, where the body repairs and rejuvenates, builds bone and muscle, and boosts the immune system? How many times do you wake up during the night? Do you wake up between 2 and 4 a.m. and have trouble falling back to sleep? You will know if you are getting enough sleep by the way you feel the next day. If you are sluggish, low on energy, and unclear in thinking, you haven't had enough good quality sleep. The lack of healthy sleep results in anxiety, depression, health problems, constant colds, and various other illnesses.

When you obtain the proper amount of sleep, your immune system stays healthy and strong. Not only that, you could actually be preventing yourself from being afflicted by dementia by getting enough of the right kind of sleep. It would be a tragedy if you suffer from the onset of dementia from a lack of sleep caused by over-worrying or stressing out over the afflicted person. Your loved one would be very happy to know that you were doing everything you could to keep yourself healthy, stress-free, and productive.

In this section, I am going to discuss ways in which you can help keep your immune system as healthy as you possibly can, along with strategies to avoid caregiver burnout. Many believe that giving away lots of love and compassion will help to keep you spiritually strong. This may be true; however, you still need to "refill" your reserves every day, especially after giving lots of your heart, soul, and time away to those who really need you. Therefore, I would like to share some ways in which you can deal with stress and replenish your soul so that you won't suffer burnout or be tempted to give up altogether.

Avoiding Burnout

"Happiness is an attitude. We either make ourselves miserable,
or happy and strong.
The amount of work is the same."
Francesca Reigler

If you are already burned out, it may be difficult to sidestep it at this point. The main idea is to treat your burnout as soon as possible. Burnout is insidious. You don't really know you are suffering it until the symptoms are too deeply entrenched, such as when you can't get out of bed or you find yourself crying easily. Even the slightest problem seems too much to handle. Don't beat yourself up with guilt if you get burned out again after treating it once or twice. It's very likely to rear its ugly head repeatedly until you wake up to the fact and the realization that you must take good care of yourself.

Even when you start feeling stronger in spirit and are emotionally healthy, there are always going to be specific things you will need to watch out for. If you notice occasional bouts of anger and depression, it's very likely you are on the borderline of burnout once again. To avoid sinking deep into depression, you must take control of your thoughts. Depression is not bigger than you are; you are bigger than it, and you can stop yourself from sliding down what appears to be a dark, slippery slope.

At the same time, don't let anger or anxiety bubble over. Stem these at their source by recognizing the point of origin. For example, anger is the outer result of a build-up of emotional pain that you haven't been able to express. If you need to release the buried pain, make the time to talk to a friend, parent, brother/sister, or counselor. Also, try sitting down in front of a computer, and begin writing. We've already talked about this in a previous chapter, and it's important to reiterate the necessity of creating the time and space for yourself to fully participate in a stress-relieving practice.

When you begin writing, write a letter to the person who hurt you. If you are feeling pain or frustration regarding the parent/elderly person that you are taking care of, write the letter to him or her.

You are not to give or send this letter at any point in time. This is just a means for you to get all of your feelings out. If you want to, strike a match to the letter and let it burn into ashes. Do this in the kitchen or bathroom sink, as a precaution.

It may sound like a simple exercise, but the purpose is to let out the pain in a safe manner. If left unattended, the pressure of the pain will build up, and the emotion will behave like hot boiling water that needs to find an outlet for its steam; otherwise, the onslaught of unrelieved pressure will cause the kettle to explode all over the kitchen floor. Don't leave it till it's too late.

Staying Healthy

"By choosing healthy over skinny,
you are choosing self-love over self-judgment.
You are beautiful!"
Steve Maraboli

Besides writing letters, journaling, going out with friends, and listening to music, it's vital to stay healthy. Staying in tip-top shape is important and can be achieved through light or medium aerobic exercise, strength training, swimming, dancing, playing tennis, or an abundance of other fun activities. Exercise is vital, and you should participate in physical activities around five times per week if possible, but commit to at least three sessions a week. Exercise keeps you healthy and strong, and helps to lift your self-esteem and feelings of well-being.

Keep your immune system strong by eating right and taking supplements. Supplements such as vitamins, minerals, and herbs provide the nutrients that your body needs. Herbal supplements are available to treat and prevent depression, stress, and can even cleanse your body of toxic substances. Detoxing is necessary when you are burdened with a bad diet and an unhealthy lifestyle.

The liver is a small organ in the body; it's often overlooked, but it has a powerful function. It cleanses us of the toxins in the air we breathe, the pollutants in the tap water and other drinks we consume, and the medications we take. If our livers are not functioning fully, we are going to feel worn down and stressed out. Cleansing the liver a couple of times per year, through any of the recommended liver cleanses will have you feeling brand new, energetic, and very healthy again. Health food stores sell pre-packaged liver detoxes that come with the required herbal supplements and nutritional support for a liver cleanse.

If you are not fully open to the idea of a thorough liver cleanse, there are specific fruits and vegetables that will assist you in mildly detoxing the liver. These include limes, lemons, grapefruit, garlic, asparagus, cayenne pepper, and spinach. Even green tea can help to keep your liver healthy. If you aren't partial to lemons and limes, squeeze a little bit into your mineral water, and drink this a few times per day.

Not only will they keep you healthy, but certain foods such as spinach, avocado, red peppers, squash, pumpkin, and salmon have high amounts of Vitamin E, which are great for your skin. This vitamin is also key to building a strong immune system, keeping the eyes healthy, and staving off heart disease and diabetes. You can keep yourself healthy with good nutrition, with foods that are easily available in the markets. Experiment for taste, and open yourself up to variety. After all, it's the spice of life!

Dealing with Stress

"All relaxation does is allow the truth to be felt. The mind is cleared, like a dirty window wiped clean, and the magnitude of what we might ordinarily take for granted inspires tears."
Jay Michelson

It is vital that you fill yourself with the love, joy, and peace of heart that's necessary to keep stress at bay. Do this upon waking every morning with an exercise of gratitude. On waking, even before you brush your teeth, count at least 10 things in your life that you are grateful for. It could be something as simple as the smell of your favorite coffee or tea, or the flowers that are blooming in your garden. Count everything, big and small, that brings a smile to your face. The more you can bathe yourself in gratitude, the more joy will arise from deep within your being. Joy keeps us young and vibrant. If you are skeptical about this, take a look at children in the playground. They epitomize joy and happiness.

Staying grounded in the present moment, and focusing on what you are doing, is a good way to fight stress. Meditation is a good practice to stay in the moment. Keep your meditation practice simple. Find a comfortable place to chill out and relax, and make sure that you can grab 15 minutes alone with no one bothering you.

How about acupuncture to relieve stress? Many people stay away from acupuncture because they are afraid of needles. However, acupuncture is a truly experiential therapy, and you "shouldn't knock it until you try it."

Acupuncture therapy helps to release calming endorphins into the blood stream and bring the body into balance. Some acupuncturists choose to apply heat to the acupressure points on the body instead of inserting needles. Regardless of the modality employed, acupuncture stimulates the flow of energy and revitalizes connective tissue, muscles, and nerves that would not be accessible by other means. A massage is very comforting and soothing. Don't defer this form of self-care till you go on vacation. Work it into your regular schedule, and you'll find that you'll be better balanced to handle the burden of caregiving.

Peace and Tranquility

Relieving stress is more about peace and tranquility of body and mind than it is about anything else. Evaluate your life to see if you have invited peace and tranquility into it. All of us tend to underestimate the power of peace. Not only does a peaceful mindset keep us sane, it gives us strength to maintain our daily schedules. When you have been chosen by the Universe to take care of someone with Alzheimer's or dementia, it's vital that you carve out for yourself a regular schedule of relaxation and rest.

Many people think that they cannot possibly relax unless they are on vacation. Please don't make that mistake. You need to take little breaks every now and then to get away from routine and to give your mind, body, and soul a refresher by doing something new.

Relaxation can take the form of daytime naps, happy hour at the local bar, an hour of yoga, reading a book, listening to music, or watching a movie. Prayer, meditating on quotes or affirmations about self-love and acceptance, or joining a local church are spiritually-based options to enhance serenity, strength, and compassion for the self and others.

Respite Care

"It is not the load that breaks you down. It's the way you carry it."
Lena Horne

Respite care simply means having someone else temporarily take care of your loved one. This is to give you a break for your own rest and relaxation, to complete chores, or to run errands. Friends and family members can easily provide in-home respite care services. Alternatively, you can hire someone or find a volunteer to help take care of your loved one while you take some time off.

You may also hire personal care or home health aides to provide grooming services, which include exercising, feeding, showering, bathing, dressing, and helping the patient with the toilet. You could also employ a separate person to help with housekeeping tasks such as laundry, cleaning, grocery shopping, and cooking. However, it may be cost-efficient to find one person who can do it all. Many provinces have free or low-cost government adult day centres, which provide a place for your loved one to get involved with others during planned activities such as art, music, and other creative programs. These centres normally provide transportation, and may even give out free meals.

Another option would be an overnight stay at a residential facility, which can be extended out to days or even weeks. This is a very secure option for those who need a long vacation. You don't have to worry about burdening family or friends for an extended amount of time. Your loved one's mental and physical health must be well taken care of, and residential facilities will provide this and everything else necessary to keep the patient safe and sound. Even though it may be more expensive, and is often not paid for by insurance, the extra cost is definitely worth your total peace of mind.

Chapter -11-

The Power of Love and Compassion

"Caregiving often calls us to lean into love we didn't know possible."
Tia Walker

Love in Action

Once you have decided to forgive and to be compassionate with yourself, it's time to make a conscious decision to love others, no matter what. Love is a choice you must make, even when you don't feel like it. Even though compassion lives in the heart, you may not always "feel" it first.

It's easy to fall in love, but it's difficult to remain in love. In order to stay in love, one must take action even when the feelings and passion have dissipated. This is the same for friendships, and for the relationships that we have with family members. When it comes to the people that we are taking care of, we must remember that action can feed emotion, and vice-versa.

If you decide to cook your mother or father dinner, even if you have had a bad day, or if they are ungrateful to you, you are going to feel good about what you have done. In this example, you can use the action to feed the feeling. You must remember to move forward in faith, believing that your compassion will be displayed and felt by those who receive and eat the meal you have prepared.

What else can you think of that demonstrates love in action? What can you do for yourself or others, even when you may not be feeling the love as strongly? Remember, when you choose to love yourself, you will automatically love others without thinking much about it. It can be as simple as taking a short break and going for a walk. We don't always feel like exercising, but when we begin moving, we feel better, stress is released, and endorphins begin floating through our bloodstream, giving us feelings of relief and well-being. It is the same for performing actions with unconditional love, without expecting anything in return.

Love Is Power

Love is not typically defined as power, but it can be experienced as such. When you sow love, you reap power. I'm referring to strength of spirit or "heart." When you wake up in the morning, do you automatically feel good? Probably not!

To get to your best, you need to make preparations. Some people might drink a cup of coffee first, take a shower, eat breakfast, and watch the news. Others may decide to meditate, pray, or read. With this love and self-care, you are going to be far more equipped to get things done.

After you have given yourself some care in the morning, you are ready to care for others. It doesn't always have to be extravagant. People believe that loving others is all about grand gestures, and nothing could be further from the truth. They get overwhelmed when they cannot live up to expectations. At this point, many people choose not to do anything at all.

When you are dealing with people who have become disabled through dementia or Alzheimer's, you need a different kind of love, something that involves you giving more and finding your satisfaction in service and care.

When you care for a family member or friend with the disease, you are bringing love to their life. You can change their lives for the better just by being available to them when they need you. Saying one positive statement can fill their entire day with joy. Giving your loved one a smile from ear to ear may be just the thing that they needed. It can touch their heart deeply.

It can be hard to remember how important we are to other people, especially if they can no longer express it the way that they once did. Sometimes it's hard to believe that you are making a difference. Life is rough. Trials and tragedies abound everywhere we look. Car accidents, cancer diagnoses, and substance abuse have taken this world over. However, we don't have to let these things rule us. We can choose to rise up above the chaos, and bring in love, light, and joy.

Will you make the choice today? Will you let your heart emit its true strength through love and compassion?

Love as a Tool

Love itself is a tool, but if you have never been taught how to love others, you must learn to love yourself first. I want to reiterate this because it's impossible to truly love others if you don't love yourself compassionately first. You must learn that gentleness, kindness, patience, and compassion are the greatest forms of love that you can show to your suffering loved one, as well as yourself. The stricken may not understand what you are saying from one moment to the next, but they will be able to connect with the feelings and emotions that emanate from your soul to theirs.

Remember that in most cases, most patients are unaware of what they are saying. Many times, you will hear them repeat the same sentence or idea over and over again. This is frustrating, even maddening, but this is also a natural thing as they move into the middle and end stages of Alzheimer's disease. Their questions may be absurd. Be patient, be kind, and remember that they cannot help it. Here, love acts as a tool to help you be patient.

Love also teaches us to laugh. Lightheartedness and laughter are great ways to keep your spirit strong, as well as to interact with your loved one. If you are having a rough day, or just a difficult time in pulling love out of your heart to give, then lighten up, crack some jokes, and laugh. People who are afflicted by this illness are nonetheless capable of feeling joy; halt any negative feelings, such as frustration or impatience, by turning toward laughter.

Watch a comedy together. Be silly. Being excellent is good, but being ridiculous can take the pressure off. Laughter is the best medicine, so take it and give it away frequently.

Choose Love, Not Anger

Do you lash out in anger, or do you channel it into constructive and open communication with another? To use anger for your good, be open with others when they hurt you or say something to upset you. Being honest and speaking out will help to heal your heart. When you are honest with others and release your pain immediately, you will feel free and lighthearted!

When someone is in the mid to late stage of Alzheimer's, they may often be confused, upset, or unaware of what is going on around them. In most cases, your forgiveness will not change anything for them, but it could change everything for you. When you forgive someone, you will be able to release the anger and pain that you feel. It does not matter what it does or does not do for them. Forgiveness is a way for you to cleanse yourself and to start over fresh.

Find Strength in the Emotional Bond

You have the ultimate power to strengthen the emotional bond between you and your loved one. At the early caregiving stage of the disease, your loved one is still able to take care of him or herself, and be willing and present to strengthen the emotional bond. However, as the disease progresses, this duty falls to you. Someone who is suffering from a degenerative disease may have the emotions dialed all the way up or down.

Love is very powerful, and you never know when you might see it. Some people think that the real tragedy of the disease is that it is so unpredictable, but every day can bring with it a glimmer of hope, one more moment, or even a handful of hours with someone who may slip back into the way that they once were. These are the brief moments when you come face to face again with the person you remember him or her to be.

Your loved one may not be able to appreciate all of the effort that you put into caretaking for him or her, but you can appreciate and reward yourself as time goes on. Caretaking is a tiring procedure, but it is one that tells you a lot about yourself, and it can show you that you are capable of a strength that you've never discovered before.

Don't delay. It is never too late, and it is never too early to start strengthening an emotional bond. Through your taking care of them physically, the emotional bonds will greatly deepen with each interaction. Your loved one may not be able to remember your face or who you are, but they will always feel your love deep within their souls. When you spend time with your loved one, companionship and communion will develop.

Real Compassion

"I cared about them. I wanted them to feel better, to live better lives. And then it occurred to me—I cared about myself. I wanted me to live a better life too. Caring about myself was allowing me to care about others."
Cate Tiernan

Sometimes it is hard to see the act of caring for someone with Alzheimer's or dementia as an act of love. Being a caretaker for someone with a serious disease is something that is very difficult, and it can become a burden. Managing the negative emotions that come with caregiving takes time and effort, but it is something that you must learn to do. Compassion is going to be one of the best tools in your arsenal when it comes to dealing with these negative feelings.

Finding compassion for others can be hard, even for the kindest people. We are not as kind as we want to be sometimes, but we can find it within ourselves to do more than we think we can. Understanding the role of compassion in this struggle, both for your parents and for yourself, is essential.

Compassion gives us armor. Instead of making us vulnerable, it makes us strong. If you have compassion and understanding, suddenly the pains of the world hurt you less. This all cycles back to compassion for yourself first. If you allow yourself to be easygoing, comfortable with yourself, and laid back, you will have no problem doing the same for others around you.

We have already talked about self-compassion and so forth, but it's always worth mentioning again. We easily forget that loving ourselves takes first priority in life, no matter what we have been called to do and take on.

Love is a great challenge, but it's also the most fulfilling action you can take. Real compassion arises within the spirit, moves out toward the soul, is felt deeply in the heart, and is seen in the eyes. The eyes are the windows to the soul. If the other person to whom you are speaking can see the compassion in your eyes, he or she will feel it deep within their heart.

When you speak with someone, truly see them. Make eye contact, and connect with them on a deep level. This is especially important for those with dementia or Alzheimer's; they may not always understand or remember what you say, but they can feel your emotions of love and compassion. They know when you are seeing them as a duty or as burden. Give them the common respect of seeing them as people.

When you are compassionate, both with yourself and with others, you will be able to create a bond where you are equals in a spiritual sense, even if you are in the relationship of caregiver and patient.

Compassion Begins with Self-Compassion

The worst thing you can do is suppress your feelings. Whether you are feeling anger, frustration, or unhappiness, remember that this is a natural outgrowth of needing to care for others.

Be honest with yourself, because the first form of true self-compassion is honesty. Admit that you need a break. Admit that you need help. Admit that you are only human and you are vulnerable to feeling stress or feeling fatigued. It is important to open up your heart and tell yourself that you need love. Everyone on this earth needs love. But those who give themselves away to others constantly need more refills of love than others.

Self-criticism is a ticking time-bomb. The path to self-love begins with accepting the fact that you are imperfect and will never obtain perfection. Laugh at your mistakes and your slip-ups, and give yourself a break! Forgive yourself, let go of your extremely high expectations, and love yourself as you are right now. You may not even live another day, so why try so hard to be something that you aren't? Be the real person you are, with all of your flaws and failings.

Drawing Boundary Lines

A big part of loving yourself is to create boundaries. It might seem a little strange that healthy love and care involves setting up limits and saying no, but it is only when we have healthy boundaries that we can care for people to our full potential.

If you too closely identify with another's needs, and submerge your own, it's very easy to give away those parts of yourself that you should keep to yourself. If you feel guilty saying no, you have no healthy boundaries. Letting someone else make decisions for you, points to an absence of boundaries. Allowing others to unconsciously dictate to you who you are and what you "should" be doing is also another clue. You have to learn when and where to draw the line. Don't be a doormat, but don't be overpowering either. This is where real balance comes in: walking the tightrope between wanting to help and to give, while taking care of yourself.

Stay Grounded

When it comes to striking a balance in your life, you must first have both feet on the ground. If you want to have compassion for others, you must have compassion for yourself, and if you want to be able to say "yes" to people, you must be able to say "no" first. We've talked about both of these things, and now we discuss how to stay grounded.

Being grounded in reality and staying in the moment is how you can ensure that you are giving people the proper care. It is easy, in caring for an Alzheimer's patient, to get caught up in the day-to-day details and trauma. It's easy to forget yourself, and to lose sight of the big picture.

Staying centered requires being truthful with yourself. It's about accepting who you are, and it's also about staying in touch with reality. Remain balanced in everything, and stay focused on the present moment, and you will have peace, confidence, and endless strength. You must remain connected to the greater world beyond your caregiving duties. It is far too easy to let yourself get swept away and to start making decisions from a flawed perspective.

Let Yourself Grow

Growth doesn't happen just because you wish it to. Self-compassion doesn't blossom in you overnight just because you read it here. Taking action is the key to growth. No person is ever emotionally and psychologically whole, and tending to someone with a serious disease can halt your growth and your development. However, the urge to grow and change remains unchanged, and if you stifle it, you will feel very upset and constrained. You are not defined by your duties, any more than your charge is confined by their disease.

Continually remind yourself to not get stressed out over the small stuff. Life happens all the time, around us and within us. If we take life too seriously, life will take us seriously and not give us any breaks. Remember to laugh, and laugh at yourself often; it is one of the best tonics you can ever have. It takes the same amount of energy to be angry as it does to laugh, so why not choose the one that will refresh your spirit and give you a boost, no matter how stressful, demanding, or uncertain the going may be?

When you let yourself stretch and grow, you can find compassion for yourself, because you are a good person who is doing something very difficult. You are more than what you do every day, and the more you are willing to commit to your own growth, the better you will be at your caregiving duties.

From Loving Yourself to Loving Others

Compassion is a coin with two sides. As you learn to love yourself, you become more capable of loving others. The power of compassion is such that the more you give of yourself, the more you have to give.

Compassion does not mean allowing people to walk all over you, and it does not mean taking more and more on yourself until you implode. Loving yourself means installing healthy limits; when you come from a place that is grounded in reality, you are ready to love others and to care for them. Caring for someone with dementia or Alzheimer's is distressing, punishing, and grinding work. You are not fully ready to do it until you have armored yourself in self-compassion; but once you have, you are ready to do the most good you can!

Don't Overcompensate

When a parent is ill with dementia or Alzheimer's, the power balance has shifted, and you may find yourself wanting to correct old wrongs. Some people view the disease as a chance for them to reconnect with a parent who was unforgiving or unloving. They might care for the loved one, hoping to earn love or forgiveness that they couldn't earn while the person was still mentally whole.

However, Alzheimer's is a difficult disease and, though it does change people, you are still dealing with the same person underneath it all. They may have forgotten many things, and they may not remember old feelings of bitterness and recrimination, but they are likely still there.

Your parent is still your parent, and no amount of loving care will change the things that happened in the past. For most people, there is no dramatic confrontation, no confession of love or forgiveness. Do not expect a catharsis from this. If you cannot care for them out of love alone, there is a serious problem. If you cannot talk to them or be open with them, make an appointment with a counselor. You may also choose to talk to a friend or family member to help you process these difficult emotions.

Another form of overcompensation stems from a lack self-confidence. You compensate for this lack by being egotistical, angry, or over-confident. You have pain and frustration that needs to be dealt with. When you behave this way, you may delude yourself into thinking that you are taking care of your loved one; but in reality, you are taking out your anger on them, either emotionally or physically. Self-compassion is key; it minimizes the need to overcompensate, and you will be able to perceive things as they actually are.

Chapter -12-

Finding Joy
While Caring for Those You Love
(How Nutrition Can Help)

"I've learned that people will forget what you said,
people will forget what you did,
but people will never forget how you made them feel."
Maya Angelou

Alzheimer's disease is progressive and, over time, it can only worsen. However, there are many things that you can do to make as much of the time that you have as you can. The onus rests on you to manage changes in thinking and behavior. Take advantage of every moment. Your loved one has only so much time, so do your best to help them enjoy what they can.

When your patient begins to decline, and especially as that decline speeds up over time, things are going to be frightening and upsetting. However, it is important to remember that life is all about balance, and that there will still be scattered moments of joy. If you have been caring for an Alzheimer's patient for a while, you know exactly what I mean; but if you are at the beginning of this journey, you may be feeling a little nervous. Remember that this is a process, and that there are going to be days where you slip up.

Interacting with Your Loved One

"We shall never know all the good that a simple smile can do."
Mother Theresa

Communicating with your loved one, before their illness, involved talking, typing, coffee dates, and other types of contact. However, when Alzheimer's sets in, the communication rules change. People with this diagnosis of Alzheimer's and dementia will use different sentence structure and formatting when speaking. They may use their hands to talk, or they may find themselves at a total loss at how to express themselves.

When communicating with someone with Alzheimer's, pay attention to their body language. They may be trying to communicate something to you but are having a difficult time finding the words. Since they cannot seem to put words together in a proper sentence, they might get frustrated and even give up. It doesn't mean that they don't need you. Be comforting and show them that you are determined to figure it out and fulfill their wants and needs as much as you possibly can.

As a caretaker, if you have never used your intuitive awareness, now's the time more than ever to do so. You must learn how to connect spiritually with your loved one. It's very simple to connect your own spirit with theirs. Relax and use your intuition. This can save you in a way that worry and stress won't. What do you think they need? How do they feel? How are they expressing themselves?

If your mind is in overload, you cannot hear what their heart is trying to tell you. Simply move your thoughts out of the way, clear your mind, and be at ease. This is the best and maybe the only way to understand what an Alzheimer's/dementia patient is trying to tell you.

Your intuition might not work very well at first, especially if you have never attempted to follow it before. Give it some time to work for you. Don't give up right away—your loved one really needs this from you, now more than ever. Let your heart shine through patience, compassion, and the integration of spirit and heart.

Be consistent in regard to your loved one's surroundings, routine, and activities. The more consistency you can offer them, the more predictably they will behave. At a time when their mental landscape is fractured and uneven, any consistency you can offer will help.

Be the leader, the one to make the decisions. People diagnosed with Alzheimer's have a very difficult time making decisions and figuring things out. You have to take on the role of "problem solver" in their lives. If they seem rebellious against your authority, just be patient and kind. Let them know that you are giving them a break so that they can have it easy, so to speak. No one that is diagnosed with Alzheimer's disease is having a good time. Be patient with them, and be willing to give them the order that they need.

Love through Good Nutrition

"The hunger for love is much more difficult to remove
than the hunger for bread."
Mother Theresa

Making sure that someone is well fed is a form of giving love. It's also a "gift" that not everyone has. If you're someone who lives off fast food and soda, this could be the most difficult aspect of taking care of someone with Alzheimer's. You don't have to feel guilty, but make sure you have a back-up plan. You can get a friend or family member to cook or somehow provide meals, or find a Meal on Wheels program to deliver the food. Either way, good nutrition is a vital component of compassionate caregiving.

If you are a compassionate caretaker, as well as a son or daughter of a patient, you most likely already know the types of foods that your loved one likes and dislikes. With a little bit of research, you'll figure out what else they need in their diet, and what they need to cut back on. We all lack certain vitamins and minerals; but for those with the disease, nutritional balance is even more important.

Many elderly people have no desire to eat because they have lost too many teeth, or because they have dentures. A reduced sense of smell and loss of taste buds are contributory factors. They may not know what they are eating because they cannot see as well as they used to. This issue can lead to being underweight, and this can be dangerous.

Since some elderly folks have a difficult time eating certain foods, juicing can be a fabulous alternative. Shakes such as Ensure or Glucerna, which are packed with vitamins and minerals, are great options for those who have a difficult time eating, or who are quickly losing weight.

Juicing is a great way to provide extra vitamins and minerals to your loved one. Juicers aren't cheap, but you might be able to find a used one, or a cheaper one through Amazon. If you aren't planning on purchasing a juicer, please make sure that they are getting plenty of fruit during the day, along with vegetables during both lunch and dinner. Fruit helps people digest their meals well, and it has natural sugars, which provides a sustained energy boost throughout the day.

Another great option is soup. Soups can be made ahead of time, and you can freeze large batches. Give soups for snack time and with dinner as well. They can be made from healthy ingredients that provide essential calories and nutrients. Soups are also very easy to make; if you are not familiar with cooking, soups are a great place to start.

If your loved one needs to gain weight, find out why they are refusing to eat. It could be the type of food, or it could be because they just don't want to eat alone. If they have lost their taste buds or sense of smell, try adding new spices and flavors to their food.

If someone else is cooking the food, ask them if they can find new recipes or add new spices. Discuss the problem with them, and see if you can come up with an alternative solution together. Losing too much weight is never a good thing for anyone, especially for the elderly who need all the strength they can get.

Supplements

Besides healthy cooking, there are also some great supplements to rejuvenate the brain of the afflicted. Alpha-lipoic acid and Acetyl I carnitine are the two most popular and powerful supplements out there, and should be taken together. Alpha-lipoic acid is an antioxidant that helps to cleanse the brain and body of undesirable and harmful toxins. Acetyl I carnitine is an amino acid that is a building block of brain cells, which can also help to prevent Alzheimer's neurofibrillary tangles (insoluble twisted fibers in the brain's cells).

You can find these supplements, along with many others, at nutrition stores and some drug stores. Folic acid belongs to the Vitamin B category and is popular among pregnant women, as well as those who need help stabilizing their nervous systems.

All of the B vitamins, which are available as a complex pill or sublingual liquid formula, are fantastic central nervous system enhancers. They help heal the DNA within the brain cells. If the Alzheimer's or dementia patient isn't taking enough of the other B vitamins, along with folic acid (vitamin B9), especially vitamin B12, it can make things worse within the brain.

Fish oil or Omega 3s are great for brain health. Omega 3 can be found in fish such as mackerel, tuna, salmon, trout, and halibut. Some people do not like seafood at all, and they can easily purchase the Omega 3 supplement. Fish oil helps to shield the brain from brain cell loss, which can be a powerful protective factor in preventing Alzheimer's altogether.

Supplements such as ginkgo biloba and ginseng are widely used among all ages to increase mental focus and improve symptoms of memory loss and mood. Ginkgo biloba doesn't prevent dementia, according to certain studies. But for those already diagnosed, at the very least it can stabilize their symptoms or even slightly improve them, by increasing blood flow to the smaller blood vessels in the brain. Just like any other prescribed medication out there, it may work for some people but not for others. It's all about trial and error. Thankfully, it's inexpensive enough that if it doesn't work, your pocket won't take a big hit.

Medications

There are 2 main types of medications that are regularly prescribed by physicians to help prevent memory loss. They include cholinesterase inhibitors, such as Aricept, Exelon, Razadyne, and Cognex, along with memantine (Namenda), to treat cognitive symptoms. Cholinesterase inhibitors help with memory, cognition, language, and normal thought processes. Doctors may also prescribe vitamin E, which is a great antioxidant that is used to cleanse the brain and body from unwanted toxins, and also protects the brain cells that are left, from wear and tear. However, high doses of Vitamin E can be dangerous, so it's absolutely vital to consult a doctor first, as it can also negatively interact with other prescriptions for blood clotting or lowering cholesterol.

Crucial Physical Exercise and Activities

Physical fitness is just as vital as good nutrition. Something called BDNF, or what is known as brain-derived neurotrophic factor, is ultra-important when taking care of or treating someone with Alzheimer's disease. BDNF causes the brain cells to grow, which is vital to a maturing brain. Exercise increases BDNF levels. When you exercise, more blood flows to the brain, which in turn prevents cognitive decline. This can slow down the progress of dementia and Alzheimer's in a big way.

Exercise can relieve depression and anxiety, lower blood sugar levels, and even fight off clogged blood vessels that cause strokes and heart attacks. Your loved one with Alzheimer's will not be able to exercise all alone, so get ready to move and have fun, as well as increase your own level of health and physical fitness! You may even be able to prevent yourself from getting Alzheimer's, if you continue to exercise, with or without your loved one!

Exercise does not have to be boring and painful. You and your loved one can start out slow if you like. Tailor your exercise expectations to what you are really capable of. Walking at a normal pace for 30 minutes per day is a basic exercise that can be done, amongst many others.

During the summer time, add a little swimming and tennis. When it's cold out in late fall and winter, stay indoors and do some aerobics, dancing, and stretching exercises. Get a membership at the YMCA and enjoy reduced fees and other perks for seniors. Check out their website at www.ymca.org. Alternatively, look into a community centre or popular local gyms.

Mental and Cognitive Fitness

You and your loved one can benefit from brain exercises just as you would from physical exercise. Any activity that involves the use of the mind/brain and the eyes, hands, and/or feet can be very beneficial for the one suffering with Alzheimer's disease. If they are capable of something, they should do it. "Use it or lose it" is the mantra of many caregivers, and it should be yours as well! Reading and writing are great daily exercises if the person you are caring for is capable of them. Crossword puzzles and other types of games that can be found in those paperback books at the drug store are not only great for cognitive fitness, but they cure boredom as well. Consider playing board games or card games such as Uno, Rummy, Yahtzee, and even Scrabble. It may be hard to believe, but watching television, playing computer games, and even playing video games such as X-Box, PS3/PS4, and Wii are also great for mental stimulation. They keep the mind engaged and active when otherwise it might be wandering.

Having regular conversations is also stimulating and helps your loved one's memories come to the surface. Older people love talking, and you can receive some amazing insights about previous eras that had interesting music, fads, and clothing trends, and so forth. They also love reminiscing about past loves and war stories. Ask them questions, be interested, and do it all in a spirit of compassion. They will appreciate you so much for taking interest in them.

Listen to music together, dance, and even sing together. These are all mentally stimulating activities, and they are very good for increased cognitive functioning. If your loved one is into arts and crafts, provide a way for them to engage with their creative side. Taking them to a day centre where they can interact with others their age and get involved with various activities is not only good mental stimulation, but it gives you a break as well.

Chapter -13-

End of Life Care

*"In the end, it's not the years in your life that count.
It's the life in your years."*
Abraham Lincoln

This journey is already difficult enough without having to consider grieving the loved one's death. But with diseases like this, being aware of the end is essential. If you are in the beginning, middle, or end stages of caregiving, be sure that preparations are made. Begin as early as possible, and involve your loved one in the planning.

There are many, many decisions to make about end of life care for your loved one with end-stage Alzheimer's. They can no longer make decisions for themselves at this point. Hopefully, this book is reaching you at the beginning stages of caregiving, so that you can involve your loved one in the planning and decisions regarding end-of-life preparations, while they are still rational. If the patient is physically sick, the type of illness will determine whether the loved one is to be transferred to a hospital or be treated at their current nursing home. Here is something to consider. The nursing home is a more familiar environment, and that may influence how the loved one bounces back or recovers from the illness. Further, the loved one is likely to get more person-to-person compassionate care in the nursing home.

One of the most difficult decisions a family has to make is how much medical treatment the loved one should be given. At some point in the illness, you may have to decide to terminate the treatment. Painful as it is, it is best to discuss advanced directives with your loved one while he or she still has the mental capacity to do so.

Delaying such a discussion means, at the end of life, the painful decision rests with you and the other members of your family. Take out the guesswork; involve your loved one fully in decision making while he or she is capable. I suggest convincing the loved one to fill out legal forms as soon as they receive a diagnosis of dementia.

The Money Problem

Financial limitations will play a big part in your ultimate decisions. Don't feel guilty if you have budgetary constraints. You can only do the best you can with what you have. Be confident in your abilities to make the right choice, and don't allow guilt to overcome you if you must make a difficult decision.

Maintain a positive attitude at all times, and be encouraging toward other family members. The last thing you and your family need during this stressful time is negativity, frustration, and stress. Everything will flow so much more easily when the atmosphere is less stressful and when everyone is united in heart and mind. Of course, there will always be dissident voices. If this is the case, present your arguments in a compassionate and encouraging manner. Give the dissenters a little extra time and space if they need it. The end-of-life decision affects everyone.

Hospice

Your healthcare provider should be your first point of query about palliative or hospice care for your loved one. Many people confuse palliative care with hospice care. Palliative care is for those who are seriously ill but are not necessarily approaching death, and hospice care is for those who have six months or less to live. Palliative care is for ill patients of any age.

An Alzheimer's patient with symptoms such as muscle weakness, digestive problems, difficult sleeping, depression, anxiety, and pain is most likely to start out with palliative care, eventually transferring over to a hospice when the prognosis turns dire.

Hospice is a compassionate form of in-home care that is covered by healthcare benefits or life insurance critical illness benefits. It's a form of palliative care, but it is only for those who are medically diagnosed as having a short time left. Once an Alzheimer's patient enters into hospice care, they are not being treated for any existing diseases. At this point, they are given comfort and pain medications so that they can end their days in as pain-free an environment as possible. This is to make them feel secure and at ease while they are transitioning into their last days of life.

Preparing for the Worst

If you already know what's coming, it's best to prepare ahead of time. The question then becomes, can one truly "prepare" for death? While you can do everything in your power to prepare for the inevitable, death always carries with it an emotional weight that is hard to understand. However, much like a hurricane, you must prepare as much as you can, and be ready to bear what comes next.

Your loved one may have different behaviors and attitudes as you approach the end together, and this may not be due strictly to Alzheimer's or dementia. The body begins to shut down, and their actions could be indicative of a need to make final resolutions with family and friends. They may have a need to forgive or be forgiven. If there is something that they want to do or complete, give them the opportunity to do so if they are still mentally and physically capable. If not, help them to let go of any guilt or pain that they might be holding onto.

During this time, your loved one might be confused, fearful, or enraged. They may not understand that they are ill and dying, and they may lash out, dissolve into tears, or get consumed by grief. Be compassionate, and be aware of your own emotional state. You are also going through a hard time, so be gentle with yourself even as you are trying to take care of your loved one.

Physical changes may include change of color, increased sleepiness, greater disorientation and confusion, along with intermittent restlessness, depression, and social anxiety. They may or may not want to be around a lot of people, even close family members. Don't force them to socialize. Give as much love and care as you can on your own, pray for the person and family, and allow your loved one to come around on his or her own.

Funeral Funds

Funeral planning is always difficult, but it needs to happen sooner rather than later. If your loved one does not have life insurance, get some immediately. Not everyone can get the same amount of life insurance, but most people can get something. Call around, conduct research, and ask questions. If he or she already has life insurance in place, call the company to find out who the beneficiaries are and how the process works when the time comes.

You and your loved one can also pay for the funeral, tombstone, and other details ahead of time. Whether they want to be buried or cremated is another idea that needs to be discussed. Remember that funeral services and wakes are meant for the ones left behind to ritually honor and remember the one who has moved on.

Ask your loved one how he or she would like to be remembered. Are there specific requests for certain prayers, scripture verses, or readings for the service? Document their wishes. Ask for favorite songs and choices of music. It is a very tough topic to be discussing while the loved one is still cognizant, but if he or she fully understands the reason behind advanced planning, it reduces the sting.

The funeral fund needs to include paying for a cemetery plot and a tombstone. Check what they would like written on the grave marker and, if possible, have it paid for ahead of time.

The Memorial Fund

"Life is pleasant. Death is peaceful.
It's the transition that's troublesome."
Isaac Asimov

A memorial fund is necessary if your loved one didn't prepare ahead of time. It may feel tacky or disrespectful to ask for help in this area, but the truth is that sometimes it is necessary. There is no shame in asking your community for help when you are in a cash crunch. Memorial funds may be requested and given ahead of time, but in other cases, they are brought up at the funeral itself or afterwards.

A memorial fund dinner is a fundraiser that sells tickets to attendees, with the money raised going toward funeral costs. Many fundraisers provide entertainment, while others include time for special readings and prayers.

Ask local restaurants, firehouses, or churches if they would be willing to provide the location at a low cost; some may be willing to offer the space for free. If you have to rent a dining hall, or a hotel conference room, contact local companies, sports teams, or other non-profit organizations to donate something special to the memorial fund in exchange for providing a venue for them to advertise. Arrange as much as you can ahead of time.

In Conclusion

Hopefully, I've given you some good ideas to implement. No one can tell you exactly what to do, not even me. As a caregiver, mentor, and author, I want to bring knowledge, wisdom, and hope to those who have loved ones with dementia and Alzheimer's disease. While I cannot tell you exactly how to heal, I want to light the way for you to find your own path.

I have felt firsthand the stress of caregiving. I have discovered how powerful love and compassion can be. Love and compassion helped me fight onerous stress. They must be nurtured and developed. You may not feel loving all the time, but in choosing to be caring and giving in service to someone who is sick, you will be infused with love. Remember that love is always a choice and, when you choose this way of life, it will give you tremendous strength during your darkest hours.

I have loved and I have lost. Losing a loved one is probably the most difficult thing on this earth. When it happens, you are riddled with pain and suffering. It cannot be avoided. The best thing you can do for yourself is to accept the loss and pass through the pain to the other side of life. When you emerge from the pain, you'll renew your love of life, but you need to first endure the pain to get to that point.

You are being beckoned to a higher life—one that you never knew was possible before you experienced death. While your loved one is being called to a new existence, so are you. It will take plenty of time, hard work, and effort, but there is more waiting for you.

Some days you will feel like giving up; on others, you will be empowered to take action. There is healing in action. There is healing in living life. Always remember that this is what your loved one wants from you. He or she doesn't want to see you paralyzed or emotionally shut down till you reach your end of days.

The more you sit back without taking action, the harder it gets in the end. This book gives you the wisdom to know where to start and how to finish. From the very beginnings of caregiving, until the day you must say goodbye, you have the tools you need. Please use them, as you will find strength—not in reading about them but in actually utilizing them. Engage with these teachings and take action!

To all families and caregivers of Alzheimer's and dementia patients, I would like to add these final words. Knowing that you have done your best at every step of the way will give you peace and joy. Also know that, while it was unexpressed, the spirits are grateful for all your unstinting and loving efforts and care.

www.ingramcontent.com/pod-product-compliance
Lightning Source LLC
Chambersburg PA
CBHW070704290526
45790CB00001B/438